Zied Arfaoui
Asma Riahi
Rahma Damak

Anxiety, depression and post-traumatic stress in post COVID-19

AF526117

Zied Arfaoui
Asma Riahi
Rahma Damak

Anxiety, depression and post-traumatic stress in post COVID-19

ScienciaScripts

Imprint

Any brand names and product names mentioned in this book are subject to trademark, brand or patent protection and are trademarks or registered trademarks of their respective holders. The use of brand names, product names, common names, trade names, product descriptions etc. even without a particular marking in this work is in no way to be construed to mean that such names may be regarded as unrestricted in respect of trademark and brand protection legislation and could thus be used by anyone.

Cover image: www.ingimage.com

This book is a translation from the original published under ISBN 978-620-6-70673-1.

Publisher:
Sciencia Scripts
is a trademark of
Dodo Books Indian Ocean Ltd. and OmniScriptum S.R.L publishing group

120 High Road, East Finchley, London, N2 9ED, United Kingdom
Str. Armeneasca 28/1, office 1, Chisinau MD-2012, Republic of Moldova, Europe
Printed at: see last page
ISBN: 978-620-7-96891-6

Copyright © Zied Arfaoui, Asma Riahi, Rahma Damak
Copyright © 2024 Dodo Books Indian Ocean Ltd. and OmniScriptum S.R.L publishing group

TABLE OF CONTENTS

INTRODUCTION

In December 2019, the emergence of a new form of coronavirus (SARS-Cov2) quickly created global confusion. A month later, the World Health Organization (WHO) declared that the outbreak of a new coronavirus disease, COVID-19, constituted a public health emergency of international concern with an increased risk of its spread to other countries around the world. Thus, in March 2020, COVID-19 was qualified by the WHO as a pandemic (1).

This new situation for the majority was the source of stress and psychological distress. The immediate impact of the pandemic on mental health was reported in extensive literature, mostly in the general population and among healthcare personnel. A number of studies carried out right from the start of the pandemic demonstrated the existence of psychological and psychiatric disorders, notably post-traumatic stress disorder and anxiety-depressive disorders (2).

However, work on these disorders in subjects with COVID-19 remains limited. And yet, these disorders could be seen post COVID-19, in the same way as former infections such as MERS and SARS.

Indeed, in a systematic review of 3559 subjects with MERS and SARS,

32.3% of subjects had post-infection post-traumatic stress disorder, 14.8% and 14.9% of cases had anxiety and depression respectively (3).

After the first year post-Covid-19, the WHO published a study showing a 25% increase in the prevalence of depression and anxiety (4). Faced with these alarming figures, several countries took action in the field of mental health.

Thus, the study of post-infection anxiety-depressive disorders and post-traumatic stress disorder, as well as the factors associated with them, is important to identify the care and support needs of those affected. This will enable the implementation of prevention and mental health intervention measures for at-risk subjects among those affected by COVID-19.

We therefore conducted this study with the aim of assessing the prevalence of post-traumatic stress and anxiety-depressive disorders in the general population with Covid-19, as well as the socio-demographic and clinical factors associated with these disorders.

METHODS

1. TYPE AND LOCATION OF STUDY

Our study took place at the La Rabta emergency department in Tunis. It was a descriptive cross-sectional study, conducted over a five-month period from January 1, 2021 to June 30, 2021.

2. STUDY POPULATION

Our study focused on a population of subjects with Covid 19 who had consulted and/or had been diagnosed with the disease.

admitted to the Rabta emergency department at the time of the study.

2.1. Inclusion criteria

We included subjects aged at least 18 and those who had contacted Covid- 19 at least one month ago.

2.2. Exclusion criteria

We have excluded :

- Subjects who interrupted the evaluation
- Subjects who did not respond to all the scales proposed for evaluation
- Subjects whose cards were unusable

2.3. Non-inclusion criteria

We have not included :

- Children and adolescents under the age of 18
- Subjects whose COVID-19 infection is less than one month old
- Subjects with sensory deficits that may interfere with evaluation
- Subjects with cognitive deficits hindering evaluation

3. DATA COLLECTION

We used a pre-established information sheet (Appendix 1) with six sections relating to :

Socio-demographic data :

- Age
- Gender

- Martial status
- Number of dependent children
- Where you live (alone, as a couple, in the family home)
- The number of people living under the same roof
- The residential zone
- Professional activity
- Socio-economic level: low if below the minimum wage; medium if between the minimum wage and four times the minimum wage, and high if above four times the minimum wage.

Somatic and psychiatric history :

- Somatic history
- History of respiratory disease (asthma, COPD, etc.)
- Personal psychiatric history
- History of consultation with a psychiatrist or psychologist
- Taking psychotropic drugs
- Family psychiatric history

Clinical data on SARS-COV infection :

- Date of Covid-19 infection
- Symptoms related to Covid-19
- Diagnostic confirmation method
- Hospitalization
- Use of respiratory assistance
- The place of isolation.
- Prescribed treatment (paracetamol / zinc / vitamin C / vitamin D / antibiotics) / Anticoagulants)
- The after-effects of the disease

Professional data related to the pandemic :

-An increase in workload compared to the pre-epidemic period

- Continuing to work while infected with Covid19
- Length of time off work
- The practice of a control PCR for the resumption of work
- The feeling of stigmatization

Assessment of pandemic-related attitudes:

Questions relating to attitudes in times of COVID-19 epidemics were identified. They concerned :

- Sources of information on the epidemic.
- Attitudes adopted to prevent infection by the Sars cov2 virus
- Attitudes adopted in the event of a psychological complaint during the epidemic.
- Recourse to psychological support and/or psychiatric consultation since the start of the epidemic.

3.1. Evaluation of psychological distress during the COVID19 epidemic.

4. MEASURING TOOLS

We used the following scales:

4.1. Patient Health Questionnaire (PHQ-9)

The *Patient Health Questionnaire* (PHQ-9) is a brief tool used to diagnose and measure the severity of depression. The PHQ-9 was developed by Drs. Robert L. Spitzer, Janet W.B. Williams and Kurt Kroenke in 1999. The PHQ-9 is shorter than many other depression screening instruments and can be self-administered. Adapted from the fourth edition of the Diagnostic and Statistical Manual of Mental Disorders (DSM-IV), the PHQ-9 includes the nine diagnostic symptom criteria used in the DSM-IV, including the two cardinal signs of depression: anhedonia and depressed mood.

Each item is evaluated on a severity scale ranging from zero to three where the respondent is asked to rate how many times each symptom has occurred in the last two weeks (0-not at all;

1-few days; 2-more than half the days or 3-almost every day), producing a total score ranging from 0 to 27.

We used the version validated in the Tunisian population. The threshold value was 10 (5).

- < 10: no depression
- 10 to 14: mild depression
- 15 to 19: moderate depression
- > 20: severe depression.

4.2. Generalized Anxiety Disorder 7: GAD-7

The GAD is a self-administered questionnaire developed by Spitzer et al (2006), based on DSM-IV-TR diagnostic criteria. This seven-item scale assesses generalized anxiety disorder over the past two weeks.

Validation of the instrument has shown that the GAD-7 is highly accurate not only for generalized anxiety disorder, but also for other anxiety disorders such as social phobia, post-traumatic stress disorder and panic disorder.

It is a screening tool that can also be used to indicate the severity of anxiety.

The GAD-7 can be self-reported or interviewed, in person or by telephone.

The questionnaire consists of seven items. Items are rated on a scale of zero to three. The maximum score is 21. The recommended threshold for estimating generalized anxiety is 10. We used the Arabic version of this scale(6). The scale presents three levels of anxiety as follows

- No anxiety: 0-4 points;
- Mild anxiety: 5-9 points;
- Moderate anxiety: 10-14 points;
- Severe anxiety: 15-21 points.

4.3. Revised event impact scale IES-R

The Impact of Event Scale-Revised (IES-R; Weiss, & Marmar, 1997) is a measure of the stress perceived by an individual in reference to a traumatic event during the previous seven days. Responses are self-reported and yield three post-traumatic symptom subscores (Reviviscence, Avoidance, Psychophysiological Activation), as well as a total post-traumatic stress disorder (PTSD) severity score. The scale exists in multiple languages. We used the Arabic version of this scale.

The IES-R consists of a list of 22 PTSD symptoms. The person indicates the intensity with which each symptom has manifested itself over the last seven days, self-reporting their response on a five-point Lykert-type scale, ranging from zero ("Not at all") to four ("Extremely"). The total IES-R score is calculated by summing the values obtained for the 22 items (scores 0-88) (7) .

The three sub-scores are the average of the item values for each factor.
(score 0-4):

- Reviviscence (8 items): 1, 2, 3, 6, 9, 14, 16, 20
- Avoidance (8 items): 5, 7, 8, 11, 12, 13, 17, 22
- Hyper activation (6 items): 4, 10, 15, 18, 19, 21

5. STUDY PROTOCOL AND PROCEDURE

Participants were recruited from the records of patients who had
consulted and/or admitted to the Rabta emergency department.

Subjects were contacted by telephone. After explaining the purpose of the study and the confidential, anonymous and non-therapeutic nature of the responses, participants were invited to complete the semi-structured questionnaire and the various scales.

The average duration of the telephone interview was 15 minutes for each participant.

To minimize observational bias, the same examiner was responsible for data collection, scale administration and data entry.

6. DATA CAPTURE AND ANALYSIS

First, we classified the data collected from the patients in our study. These data were then coded and entered into SPSS statistics 25 statistical analysis software.

The study comprised two stages: a descriptive study, followed by an analytical study.

6.1. Descriptive study :

We calculated simple frequencies and relative frequencies (percentages) for qualitative variables, and means and standard deviations for quantitative variables.

6.2. Analytical study

The study was carried out using Pearson's Chi-square test for validity.
and Fisher's exact test.

The study of the relationship between the quantitative variables was carried out using the Pearson "r", linear fit curves and coefficient of determination "R^2". The significance level was 0.05.

6.3. Multivariate study

We performed a binary regression to determine the factors associated with antidepressive and post-traumatic symptomatology while controlling for confounding variables.

7. ETHICAL CONSIDERATIONS

The nature of the study and the purpose of our research were clearly explained to each patient. No patient refused to answer the questionnaires. Written consent, shared in the form of an online form, was obtained by participants who had an internet connection. For the others, oral consent was obtained over the telephone. The aim was to reassure the interviewee that there would be no negative impact on his or her care, and that no personal information would be collected. Anonymity, confidentiality and patient privacy were respected.

We referred patients who had been identified as having an anxiety-depressive disorder
post-traumatic stress disorder to a specialist consultation.

We hereby declare that we had no conflicts of interest.

8. BIBLIOGRAPHIC SEARCH

This search was developed using the Pubmed, science direct, scholar google databases using the following terms "Depression, Anxiety, Post-traumatic stress disorder, CoV-SARS, Questionnaires".

RESULTS

A total of 120 patients infected with SARS-Cov2 were included in our study.

1. DESCRIPTIVE STUDY

1.1. General population characteristics

1.1.1. Age

The mean age of our study population was 57±13 years with extremes ranging from 19 to 82 years (**Figure 1**).

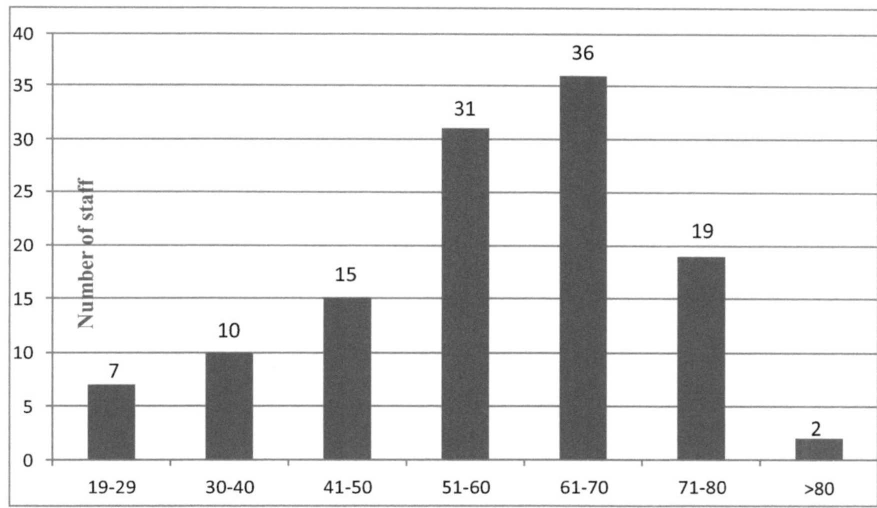

Figure 1: Age distribution of participants

1.1.2. Type

Our sample comprised 46.7% women (n=56) and 53.3% men (n=64). with a sex ratio of 1.14.

1.1.3. Martial status

Patients in a couple relationship represented 71.7% of the study population. (n=86) versus 8.3% (n=10) who were single (figure2).

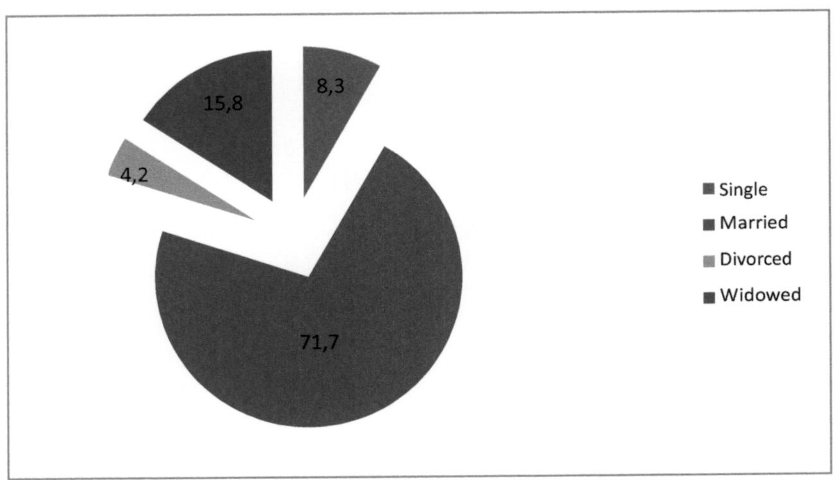

Figure 2: Breakdown of participants by martial status

1.1.4. Habitat

Fifty-eight percent (n=70) of patients lived in urban areas (figure3).

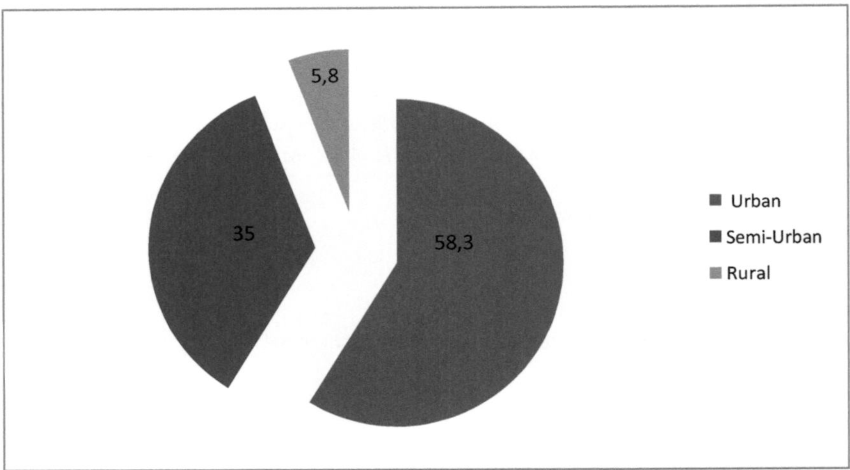

Figure 3: Distribution of respondents by habitat

More than half (n=71; 59.2%) lived with more than one person in the same household. Thus sixty-two percent had dependent children. (figure4)

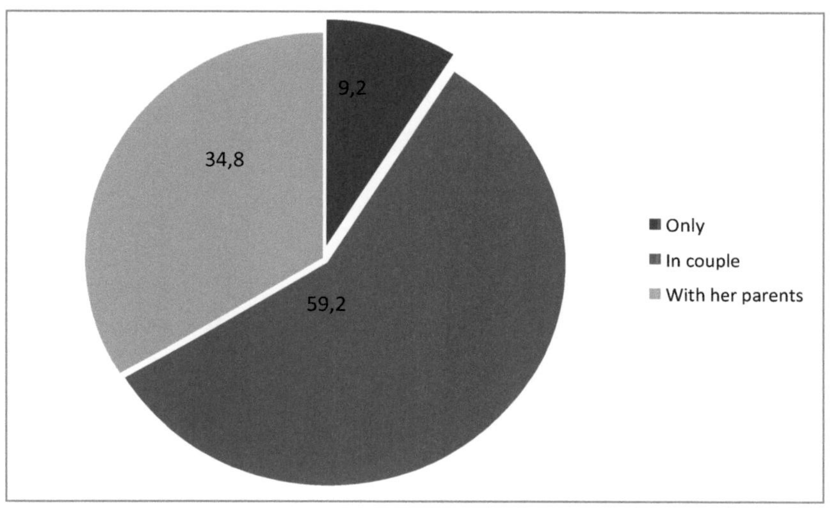

Figure 4: Breakdown of participants by number of people living under the same roof

1.1.5. Level of education :

Sixty-two percent of patients were educated. (figure5)

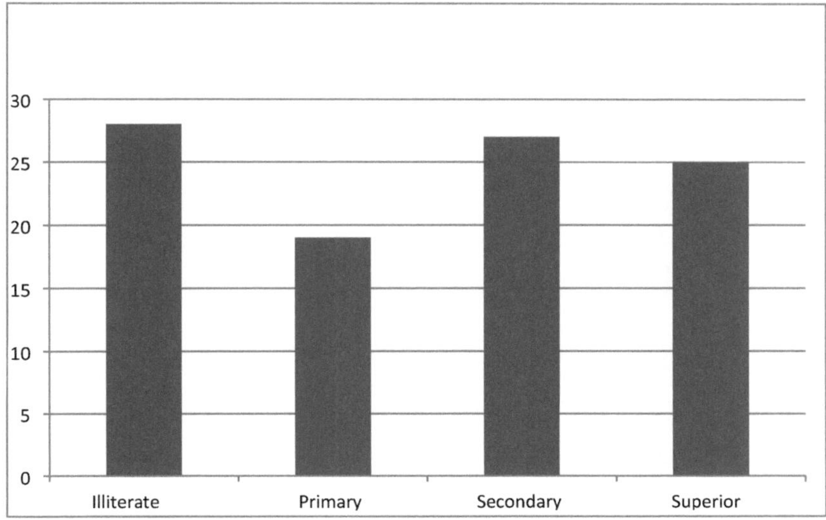

Figure 5: Distribution of participants by level of education

1.1.6. *Professional activity:*

Unemployed subjects accounted for 16.7% (n=20). Twenty-nine percent were retired (figure6).

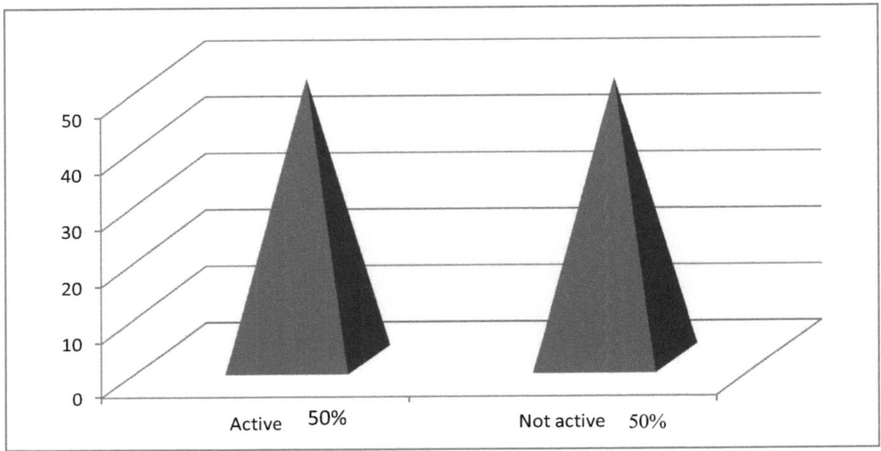

Figure 6: Breakdown of participants by occupation

1.1.7. *Socio-economic level :*

Forty-three percent (n=51) of patients had a low socioeconomic level, with a monthly income of less than 500 dinars.

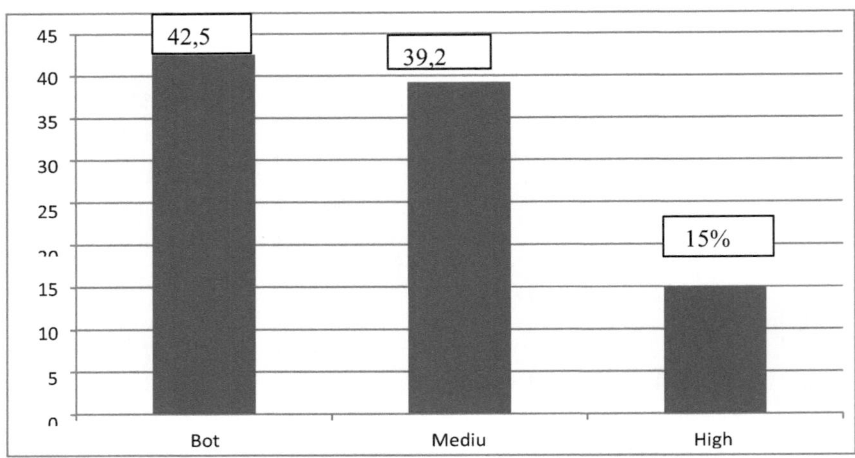

Figure 7: Distribution of participants by socio-economic level

1.1.8. Pathological history

1.1.8.1. Somatic history

Fifty-seven percent of our patients had a somatic history. The somatic histories are shown in figure 8.

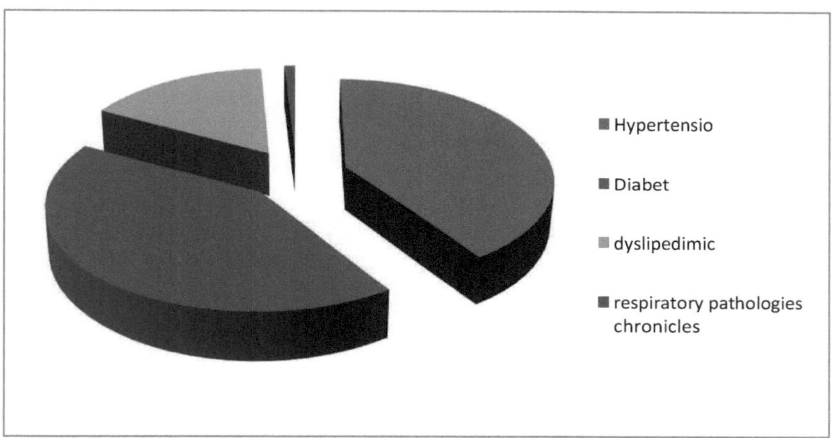

Figure 8: Distribution of patients by somatic history

1.1.8.2. Psychiatric history :

Seven percent of our patients (n=9) had a personal psychiatric history, and fifteen percent had a family psychiatric history.

1.2. Clinical features associated with Covid-19 infection:

1.2.1. Means of diagnosis :

The diagnosis of COVID-19 was confirmed by PCR in all participants. Only forty-eight percent of our patients had undergone a thoracic CT scan in the emergency department.

1.2.2. Symptomatology:

In 50% of cases (n=60), the reason for consultation was dyspnea and cough. Twenty-five percent had consulted for febrile asthenia, while twenty-one percent had consulted for digestive symptoms such as diarrhea and vomiting. (figure9)

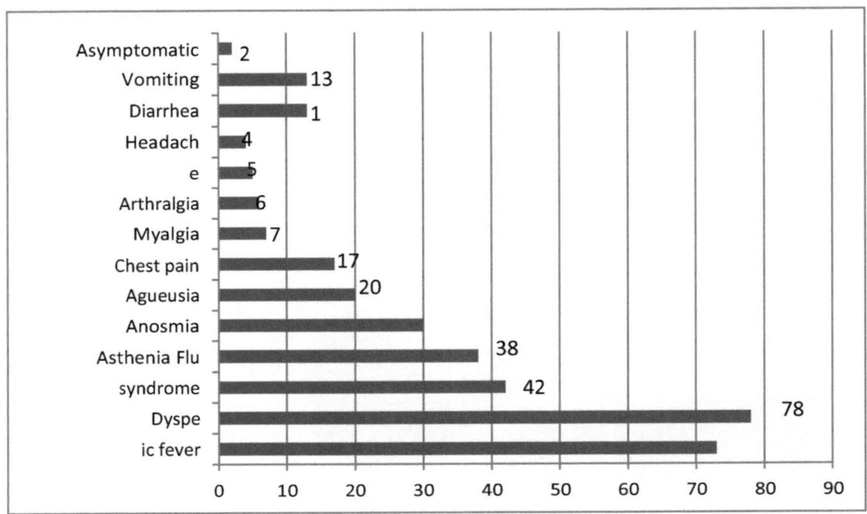

Figure 9: Distribution of patients by symptoms

1.2.3. Support

1.2.3.1. The need for hospitalization

Seventy-four percent (n=89) required hospitalization in dedicated Covid-19 wards.

Forty-one percent (n=49) of our hospitalized patients required high-concentration mask oxygen therapy. Only one patient was intubated (figure10).

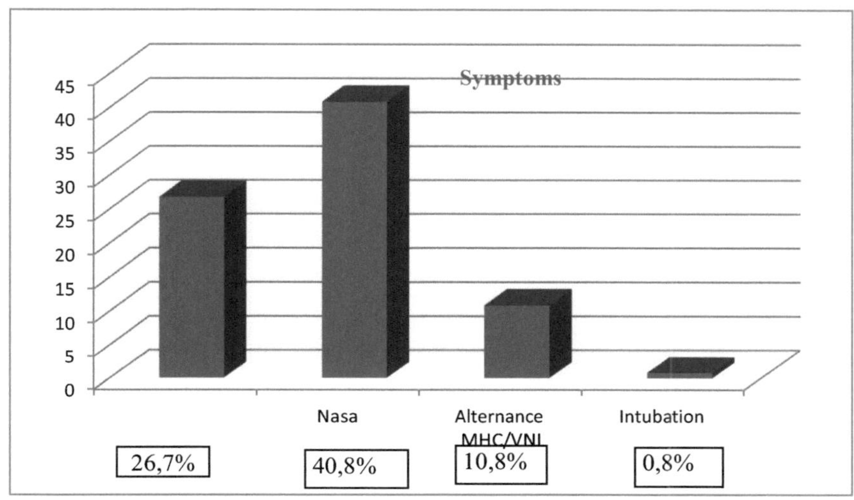

Figure 10: Distribution of patients by respiratory assistance use

1.2.3.2. Covid-19 sequelae

Over thirty percent presented a post-covid syndrome of asthenia.

Figure 11 shows the distribution of the various sequelae reported by patients.

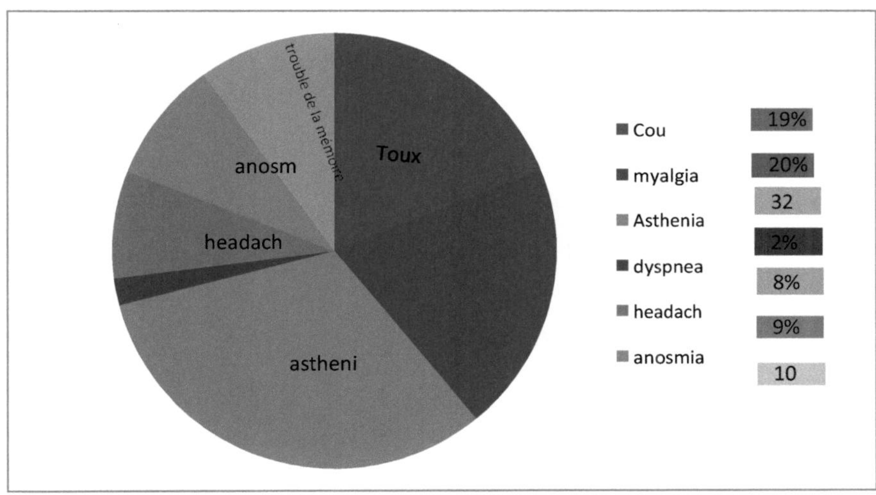

Figure 11: Distribution of participants by Covid-19 sequelae

1.2.4. Rest and return to work

1.2.4.1. Feeling of stigmatization

Seventy-five percent (n=88) had felt stigmatized for having had Covid-19 (**Figure 12**).

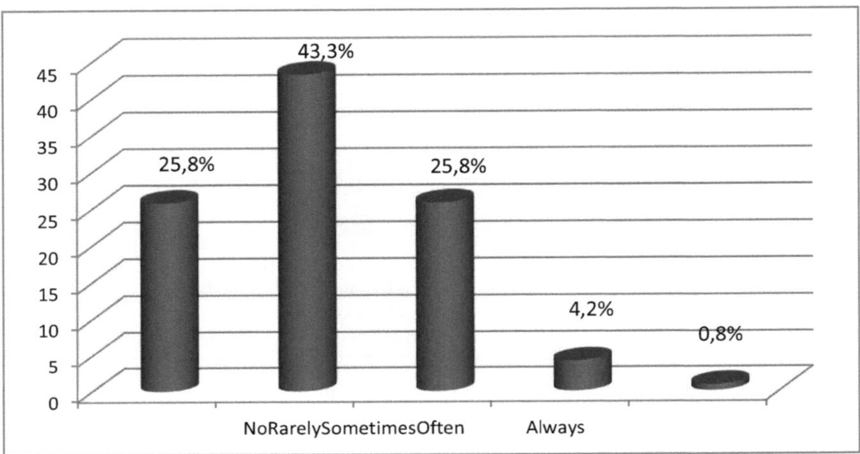

Figure 12: Distribution of participants according to their feelings of stigmatization

1.2.4.2. Stopping work

Only four percent (n=5) were teleworking while infected with Covid.

Forty percent had been on leave for between 11 and 15 days. Thirty-seven percent were discharged for more than 20 days. No patient was discharged for less than ten days.

1.3. Professional data during the pandemic

1.3.1. Working conditions and workload

Fifty-seven percent (n=68) of workers had experienced an increase in workload compared with the pre-epidemic period.

1.3.2. Pandemic behavior (before infection)

a. Hygiene and protection measures :

Fifty-seven percent (n=69) reported regular use of hygiene and protection measures in their daily activities (figure 13).

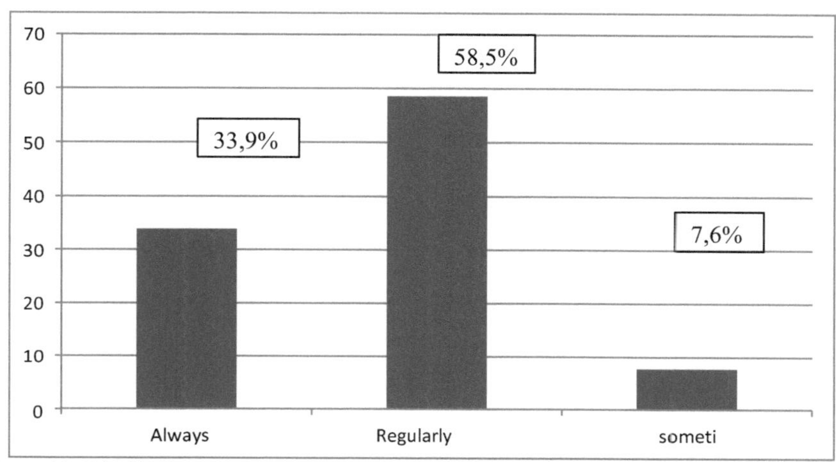

Figure 13: Distribution of respondents by hygiene and protection measures

b. The rules of physical distance :

Sixty-seven percent (n=81) regularly used the physical distancing rules.

in the workplace/on a daily basis (figure 14).

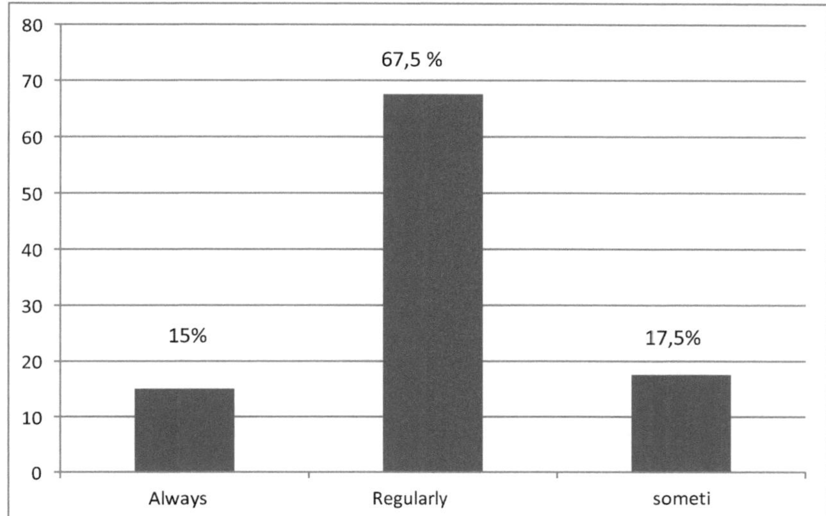

Figure 14: Distribution of respondents according to physical distancing rules

c. ***Special housing arrangements :***

Forty-four percent (n=53) had made regular housing arrangements. during the pandemic (figure 15).

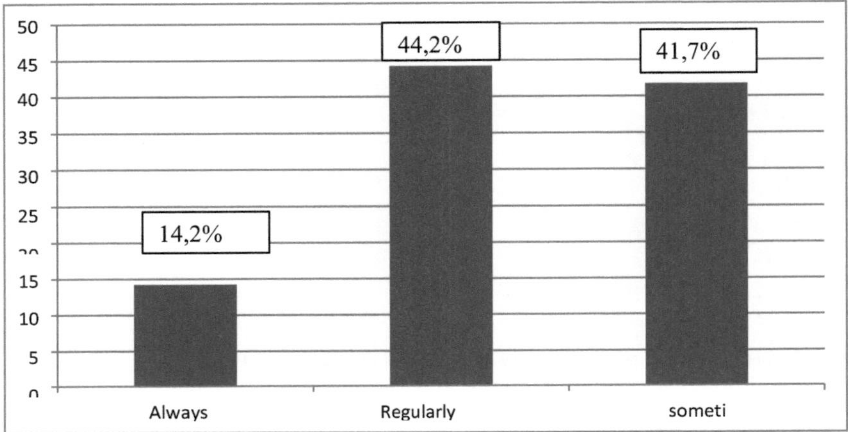

Figure 15: Distribution of respondents by special accommodation Sixty percent (n=71) had reduced their social/family contacts (figure16).

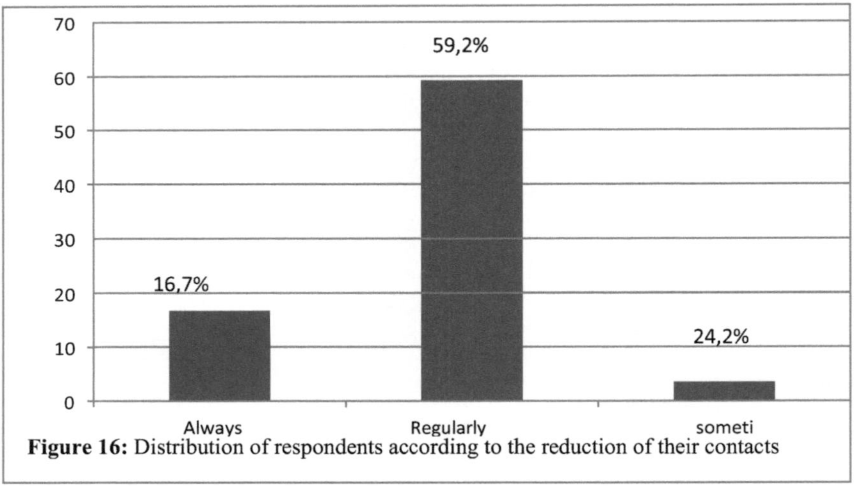

Figure 16: Distribution of respondents according to the reduction of their contacts

1.3.3. Source of information during the pandemic :

Eighty patients (66.6%) used social networks and multimedia as a personal source of information during the pandemic. Only one patient answered "I don't want to know".

Sources of information on the COVID-19 epidemic are shown in figure 17.

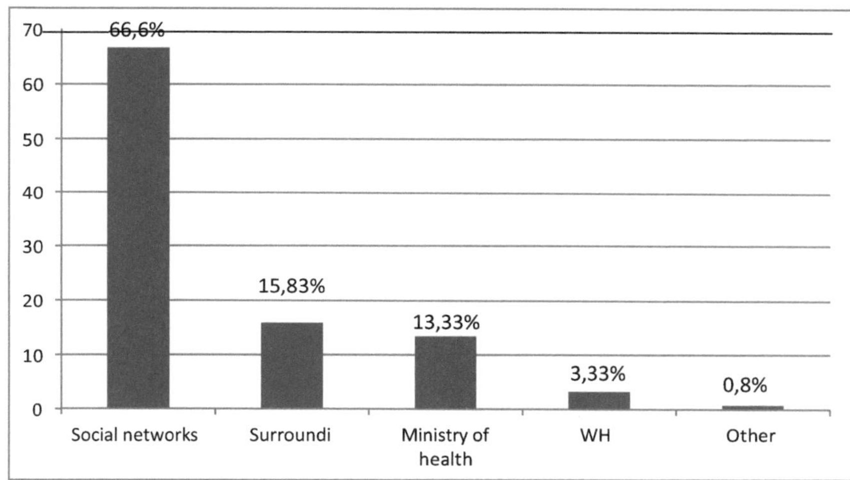

Figure 17: Distribution of respondents by source of information used during the pandemic

1.3.4. Psychological support

Sixty percent said they needed psychological support. Over half the patients did not know what to do if psychological distress occurred (n=80). Twenty-five patients said they would stay at home, ten said they would consult an emergency room or a psychologist/psychiatrist, and five said they would contact a relative.

1.4. Prevalence of anxiety-depressive disorders in the study population :

a. Prevalence of depressive symptoms (PHQ-9) :

The mean PHQ-9 total score was 14, with a minimum of zero and a maximum of 27. More than half the participants showed depressive symptoms.

The distribution of the population according to the severity of depressive symptoms is as follows

shown in Figure 18.

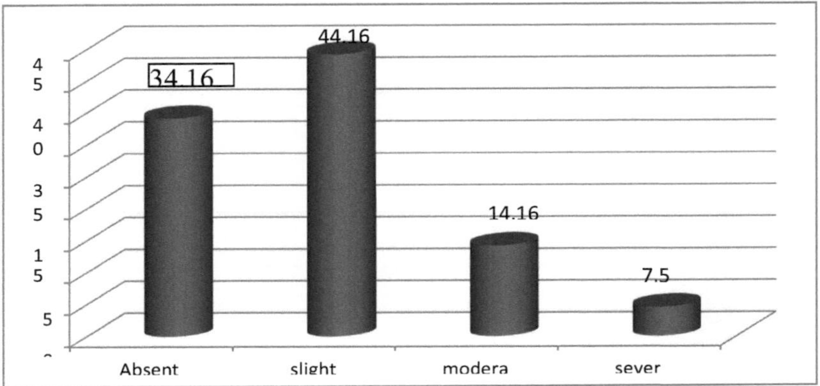

Figure 18: Distribution of participants by depressive symptomatology (PHQ-9)

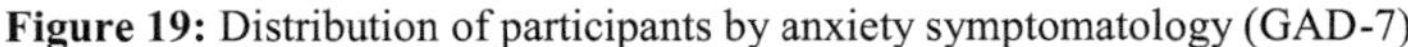

b. Prevalence of anxiety symptoms (GAD-7)

The mean GAD-7 total score was 13, with a minimum of zero and a maximum of 21. Anxiety symptomatology was noted in 116 participants. The levels of anxious symptomatology are shown in figure19.

Figure 19: Distribution of participants by anxiety symptomatology (GAD-7)

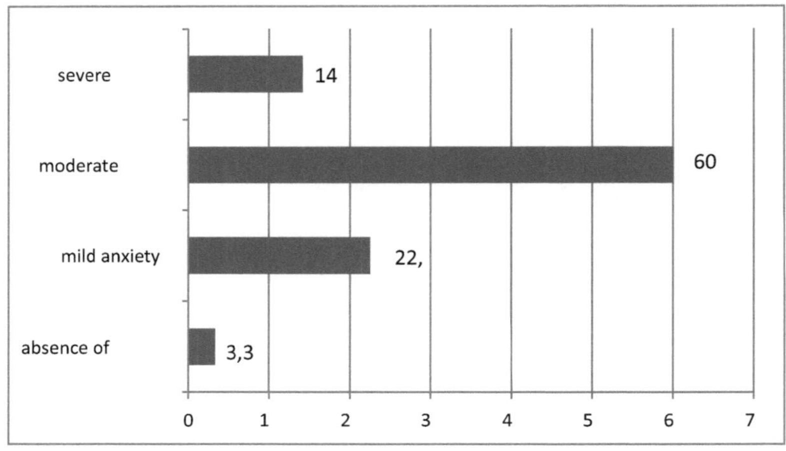

1.4.1. Prevalence of post-traumatic symptoms (IES-R)

The mean total IES-R score was 28, with a minimum of 0 and a maximum of 88. Mild symptomatology was noted in 45.83% of patients (figure 20). Table I represents the different scale scores.

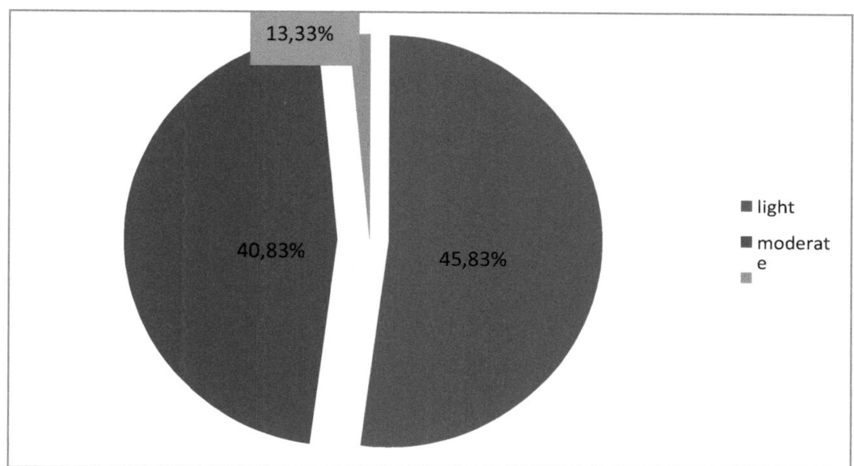

Figure 20: Distribution of participants by IES-R symptom rating

Table I: Summary of IES-R item scores

	Median	Intervals
Reviviscence	14	[0 - 23]
Avoidance	14	[0 - 25]
Hyperactivation	10	[0 - 18]
IES-R score	40 ,5	[0 - 82]

1.4.2. Co-morbidity Post-traumatic stress disorder and anxiety-depressive disorder :

Forty-six percent of patients with PTSD had mild anxiety-depressive symptomatology, 40% had moderate anxiety-depressive symptomatology and 14% had severe anxiety-depressive symptomatology.

2. ANALYTICAL STUDY

2.1. Relationship between depressive symptomatology and the characteristics of the study population

2.1.1. Relationship between depressive symptomatology and general characteristics of participants

a. Univariate analysis :

The PHQ-9 score was significantly higher in participants aged over 40, male, illiterate and those living in urban areas (Table II).

Table II: Variation in PHQ-9 score according to participants' general characteristics

Caractéristiques générales		PHQ-9 Moyenne [Intervalles]	P *
Age	≤ 40 ans	9 [1-18]	0,000
	> 40 ans	10 [0-19]	
Genre	Homme	10[1-19]	0,007
	Femme	9[0-18]	
Statut martial	Non marié	9[0-17]	0,118
	Marié	9[1-19]	
Nombre d'enfants	Pas d'enfants	9,5[0-17]	0,224
	1 enfant ou plus	9[1-19]	
Activité professionnelle	Au chômage	7[1-18]	0,409
	Retraité	10 [0-19]	
	Active	9[1-17]	
Niveau d'éducation	Analphabète	8,5[0-15]	0,032
	Primaire	9[2-16]	
	Secondaire	10[1-19]	
	Supérieur	9,5 [1-18]	
Habitat	Seul	7[3-17]	0,188
	En famille	9 [0-19]	
Zone d'habitat	Rurale	8[0-16]	0,048
	Urbaine	9,5[1-19]	
Niveau économique	Bas à moyen	9 [0-19]	0,654
	Elevé	11[5-17]	
ATCD somatiques	Non	10 [1-19]	0,437
	Oui	9[0-18]	
ATCD	Non	9 [0-19]	0,

personal psychiatric problems	Yes11 [6-16]	436

b. ***Linear regression :***

In addition, we found a moderately positive correlation between PHQ-9 score and patient age (p=0.000, β =0.417) (figure 21)

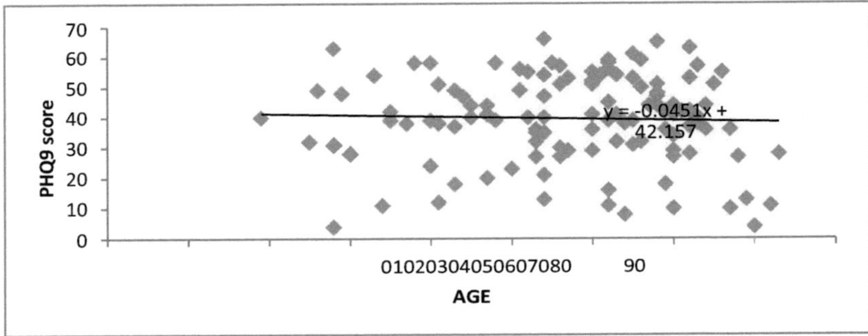

Figure 21: Correlation between PHQ-9 score and patient age

Similarly, a significant correlation was observed between gender and PHQ-9 score (p=0.016, β=-0.205) (figure 22).

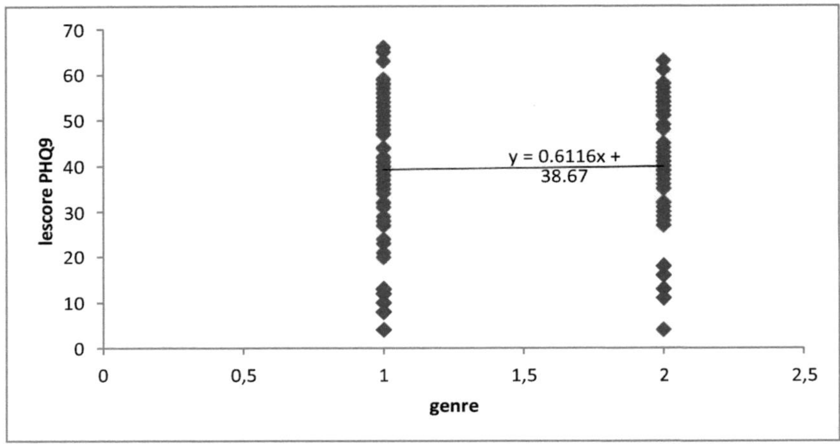

Figure 22: Correlation between PHQ-9 score and patient gender

2.1.2. Link between depressive symptomatology and clinical features related to covid-19 :

The PHQ-9 score was significantly higher in participants with sequelae following their SARS-Cov2 infection (p<0.001) (**Table III**).

Table III: Variation in PHQ-9 score according to care characteristics during the pandemic

		PHQ-9 Average [Intervals]	P
Hospitalization No 6[0-15]	Yes 11[1-19]		0,147
Respiratory assistance	No Yes	5[0-14] 11[1-19]	0,383
Sequels	Absent Present	0,5[0-1] 9[1-19]	< 0,001

2.1.3. Link between depressive symptomatology and perception during the pandemic :

Table IV: Variation in PHQ-9 score according to perception during the pandemic

		PHQ-9 Average [Intervals]	P
Source of information	ministry of health official website OMS social networks multimedia family	10 [6-15]	0,083
		12,5[4-18]	
		9[1-17]	
		9[1-17]	
		9[0-14]	
Stigmatization	Yes	9[0-15]	0,415
	No	9[0-15]	
Work being infected	No	11[1-18]	0,157
	Yes	9[6-14]	
Duration of work stoppage	< 15 days	9[1-16]	0,031
	≥ 15 days	11[1-18]	

2.1.4. Link between depressive symptomatology and pandemic behavior

The PHQ-9 score was significantly higher among participants who expressed a need for psychological support during the pandemic (p=0.002) (**Table V**).

Table V: Variation in PHQ-9 score according to pandemic behavior

Behaviour in the face of the pandemic	PHQ-9 Average [Intervals]		**P**
Use of protective equipment	Always	9[1-15]	0,091
	Not always	10[0-19]	

Cover mouth when coughing	Always	9[1-17]	0,511
	Not always	10[0-19]	
Application of distancing rules	Always	11[2-16]	0,129
	Not always	9[0-19]	
Special housing arrangements	Always	12[1-16]	0,552
	Not always	9[0-19]	
Reduced social contact	Always	10,5[1-17]	0,195
	Not always	9[0-19]	
Need for psychological support	No	7[0-14]	0,002
	Yes	11[1-19]	

*: Mann Whitney PHQ-9: Patient health questionnaire-9

1.1. Relationship between anxiety symptomatology and general characteristics of the study population (GAD-7)

1.1.1. Link between anxiety symptomatology and participants' general characteristics

a. Univariate analysis :

The GAD-7 score was significantly higher in participants aged over 40, illiterate and those living in urban areas (Table VI).

Table VI: Variation in GAD-7 score according to participants' general characteristics

General features	GAD-7 Average [Intervals]		P
Age	≤ 40 years	10[1-16]	**0,000**
	> 40 years	11[0-19]	
Type	Men	11[1-19]	0,088
	Woman	11[0-16]	
Martial status	Non marié	10[0-18]	0,327
	Mari	11[0-19]	
Number of children	Pas children	11[0-19]	0,275
	1 child or more	11[0-17]	
Education level	Illiterate	11[0-15]	**0,006**
	Primary	11[6-19]	
	Secondary	11[0-16]	
	Superior	12[1-17]	
Professional activity	Active	10[0-17]	0,260
	Retirement	11[0-19]	
	Unemployment	11,5[1-16]	
Habitat	Only	11[7-16]	0,818
	In the family	11[0-19]	
Housing zone	Rural	11[0-15]	**0,005**
	In the family	11[0-19]	
Economic level	Low to medium	11[0-19]	0,433
	High	12[0-17]	
Somatic history	No	11[0-19]	0,173
	Yes	11[0-18]	
Personal psychiatric history	No	11[0-19]	0,494
	Yes	12[0-14]	

ATCD: antecedents * : Mann Whitney GAD-7: Generalized Anxiety Disorder Scale

b.Linear regression :

A positive correlation was observed between the GAD-7 score and patient age (p=0.000 ; β=0.502) (Figure 23).

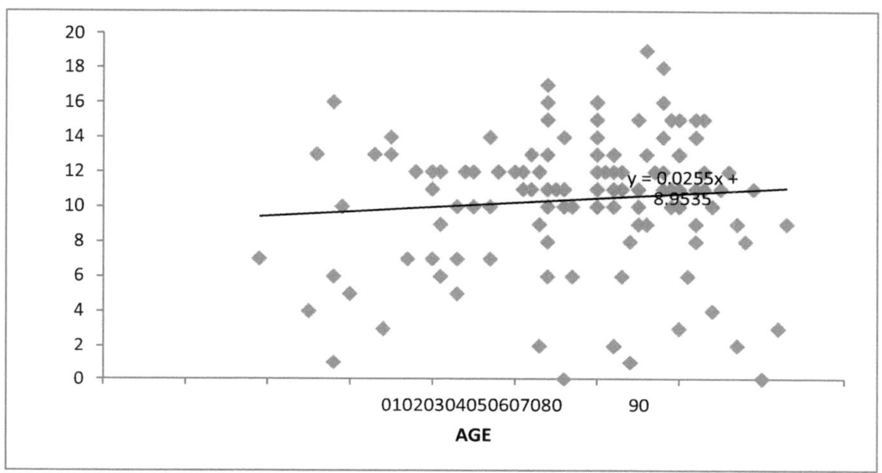

Figure 23: Correlation between GAD-7 score and patient age

1.1.2. Link between anxiety symptomatology and management during the pandemic

The GAD-7 score was significantly higher in participants with sequelae following their infection (p=0.001) and those who were hospitalized (p=0.006) (**Table VII**).

Table VII: Variation in the GAD-7 score according to care characteristics during the pandemic

		GAD-7P Average [Intervals]	P
hospitalization	**No**	9[0-14]	0,006
	Yes	12[1-19]	
Respiratory assistance	**No**	8[0-14]	0,383
	Yes	12[1-19]	
Sequels	Absent	0,5[0-1]	0,001

	Present	11[0-19]	

GAD-7: Generalized Anxiety Disorder Scale

1.1.3. The link between anxiety symptomatology and perception during the pandemic :

Subjects who felt stigmatized had significantly higher anxiety scores (Table VIII).

		GAD-7 Average [Intervals	P
Source of information	ministry of health official	11,5[0-16]	0,736
	website OMS social	12,5[4-18]	
	networks multimidia	11[1-18]	
	family	11[0-19]	
Stigmatization	Oui	11[1-19]	**0,022**
	No	9[0-15]	
Work being infected	No	11[0-19]	0,382
	Oui	12[5-14]	
Duration of work stoppage	< 15 days	8[0-14]	0,002
	≥ 15 days	12[5-19]	

1.1.4. Behaviour in the face of the pandemic

The GAD-7 score was significantly higher among participants who expressed a need for psychological support during the pandemic (p=0.005) (**Table IX**).

Table IX: Variation in GAD-7 score according to pandemic behavior

Behaviour in the face of the pandemic		**GAD-7** Average [Intervals]	**P**
Use of protective equipment	Always	10,5[0-19]	0,180
	Not always	11[0-18]	
Cover mouth when coughing	Always	11[2-17]	0,704
	Not always	11[0-19]	
Application of distancing rules	Always	11[0-14]	0,476
	Not always	11[0-19]	
Special housing arrangements	Always	11[1-16]	0,836
	Not always	11[0-19]	
Reduced social contact	Always	12[2-16]	0,680
	Not always	11[0-19]	
Need for psychological support	No	10[0-16]	**0,005**
	Yes	12[0-19]	

*: Mann Whitney GAD-7: Generalized Anxiety Depression Scale

1.2. Link between post-traumatic symptomatology and general population characteristics

1.2.1. Relationship between post-traumatic symptomatology and general characteristics of participants

a. Univariate analysis :

The IES-R score was significantly higher in participants aged over 40.

and illiterate people (**Table X).**

Table X: Variation in IES-R score according to participants' general characteristics

General features		IES-R Average [Intervals]	P *
Age	≤ 40 years	39 [4-63]	**0,000**
	> 40 years	41[4-66]	
Type	Men	40[4-66]	0,550
	Woman	41[4-63]	
Martial status	Unmarried	37,5[4-66]	0,583
	Married	42[4-63]	
Number of children	No children	40,5[4-66]	0,224
	1 child or more	40,5[4-63]	
Professional activity	Unemployed	35,5[4-63]	0,541
	Retired	42[4-65]	
	Active	40[11-59]	
Education level	Illiterate	42[4-63]	**0,009**
	Primary	38[13-65]	
	Secondary	44[18-66]	
	Superior	40,5 [4-63	
Habitat	Seul	34[27-66]	0,887
	In the family	41[4-65	
Housing zone	Rural	39[4-59]	0,233
	Urban	42[10-66]	
Economic level	Low to medium	39,5[4-66]	0,778
	High	47[10-59]	
Somatic history	No	40[4-66]	0,848
	Yes	4,5[4-63]	
Personal psychiatric history	No	4,5[4-66]	0,340
	Yes	39[13-53]	

ATCD : Antecedents * : Mann Whitney IES R: Event Impact Scale

Linear regression :

A positive correlation was found between the IES-R score and patient age (p=0.000 ; β=0.379) (**Figure 24**)

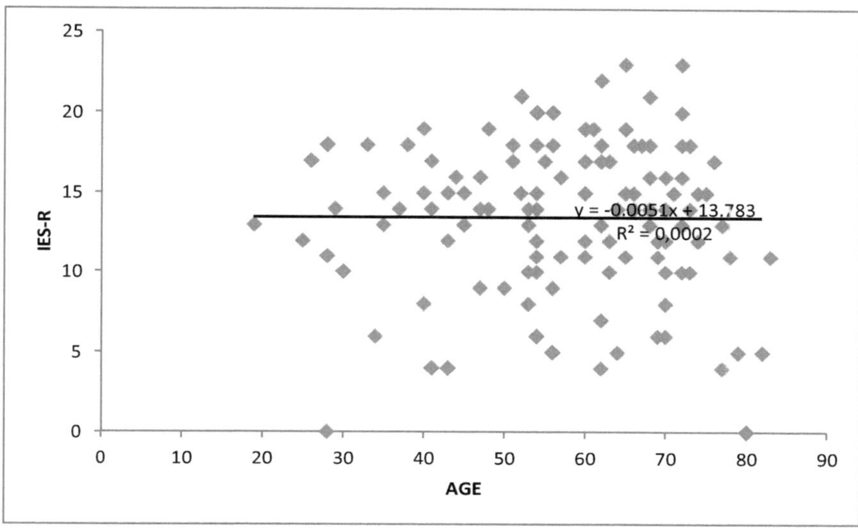

Figure 24: Correlation between IES-R score and patient age

1.2.2. Link between post-traumatic symptomatology and management during the pandemic

a. Univariate analysis :

The IES-R score was significantly higher in participants who used respiratory assistance (**p=0.028**) (Table XI)

Table XI: Variation in the IES-R score according to care characteristics during the pandemic

		IES-R Average [Intervals]	P
Hospitalization	No	28[4-54]	0,182
	Yes	44[8-66]	
Respiratory assistance	No	28[4-54]	**0,028**
	Yes	44[8-66]	
Sequels	Absent	4[4-4]	

	Present	41[8-66]	

* : Mann Whitney IES R : Event impact scale

b. Linear regression :

A significant correlation was found between the IES-R score and respiratory assistance (p=0.012, β=0.379) (figure25).

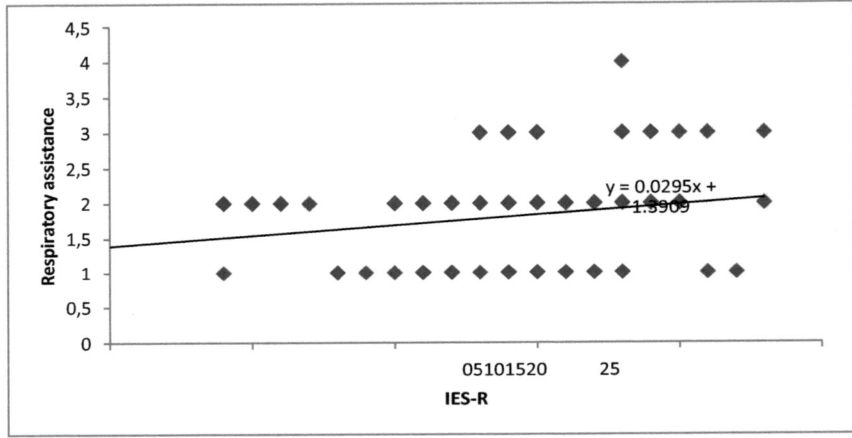

Figure 25: Correlation between IES-R score and respiratory assistance.

1.2.3. The link between post-traumatic symptomatology and perception during the pandemic :

IES-R was significant in patients rested for more than 15 days.

(p=0.014) (Table XII).

Table XII: Variation in IES-R score according to perception 1 during the pandemic

		IES-R Average [Intervals]	P
Source of information	ministry of health official WHO website	43,5[10-59]	0,384
	social networks	46,5[29-63]	
	multimedia	40[4-66]	
	family	42[4-63]	
Stigmatization	Non	41[4-66]	0,707
	Yes	38[4-63]	
Work being infected	Non	42[8-66]	0,276
	Yes	29[23-44]	
Duration of work stoppage	< 15 days	30[8-58]	0,014
	≥ 15 days	49[13-66]	

1.2.4. Link between post-traumatic symptomatology and behaviors in the face of the pandemic:

The IES-R score was significantly higher among participants who expressed a need for psychological support during the pandemic (p=0.005) (**Table XIII**).

Table XIII: Variation in IES-R score according to pandemic behavior

Behavior in the face of the pandemic		**IES-R** Average [Intervals]	P
Use of protective equipment	Always	40[10-59]	0,720
	Not always	41[4-66]	
Cover mouth when coughing	Always	42[10-59]	0,673
	Not always	39[4-66]	
Application of distancing rules	Always	40,5[10-59]	0,886
	Not always	40,5[4-66]	
Special housing arrangements	Always	41[4-54]	0,124
	Not always	40[4-66]	
Reduced social contact	Always	52[13-66]	0,325
	Not always	39[4-65]	
Need for psychological support	No	35[4-61]	**0,005**
	Yes	45,5[4-66]	

DISCUSSION

1. Main results :

We conducted a cross-sectional study in the emergency department of the Rabta Hospital in Tunis to estimate the prevalence of anxiety-depressive symptoms and post-traumatic stress in a population of patients who had contracted Covid-19 at least one month previously, and to identify the sociodemographic and clinical factors associated with these disorders.

Our sample of 120 patients comprised 56 women and 64 men, giving a sex ratio of 1.14. The average age of the subjects was 57 ±13 years. Fifty percent of patients were unemployed and 42.5% had a low socioeconomic status.

In terms of clinical characteristics, 74% of subjects had required hospitalization in Covid-19 wards, 40% of whom had used a high-concentration mask. One month after their illness, 32% of subjects had post-Covid-19 sequelae consisting of asthenia (25%), myalgia (20%) and cough (19%).

Regarding perception during the Covid-19 pandemic, 74% had felt stigmatized because they had had Covid-19. Fifty-seven percent of workers had experienced an increase in workload compared to the pre-epidemic period.

The source of information on the COVID-19 epidemic was social networks and multimedia. in 66% of cases.

In the event of psychological distress, 72% said they didn't know what to do. Furthermore, 60% expressed a need for psychological support, and only 5% had consulted a psychiatrist at the start of the epidemic.

The prevalence of depressive, anxiety and post-traumatic stress symptoms was 65.84%, 96% and 52.2% respectively.

In univariate analysis, age over 40, male gender, being illiterate, living in an urban area, having sequelae of the disease, being off work for more than 15 days and needing psychological support were significantly associated with depressive symptomatology with $p=0.000$, $p=0.007$, $p=0.032$, $p=0.048$, $p<0.001$, $p=0.031$, $p=0.002$ respectively.

In linear regression, age and gender were the independent predictors of depressive symptomatology, with $p<0.001$ and $p=0.016$ respectively.

We found a statistically significant association, in univariate analysis, between anxiety symptomatology and the following variables: age over 40 ($p=0.000$), level of education (p=0.006), area of residence (p=0.005), hospitalization (p=0.006), having sequelae of the disease (p=0.001), feeling of stigmatization (p=0.022), length of time off work (p=0.002), and need for psychological support (p=0.005). In linear regression, age over 40 was the only independent predictor of this symptomatology, with p<0.001.

In univariate analysis, post-traumatic stress symptomatology was significantly associated with the following variables: age (p=0.000), level of education (p=0.009), use of respiratory assistance (p=0.028), length of time off work (p=0.014), and need for psychological support (p=0.005). In linear regression, age and use of respiratory assistance were the independent predictors of this disorder, with p<0.001 and p=0.012 respectively.

2. Interest and limitations of the study:

The first limitation of this study was the sample size. Although recruitment was spread over a six-month period, it was smaller than expected. In addition, we conducted a study at a single Covid center. The small sample size and monocentric nature of the study made it difficult to generalize our results to the wider population.

The second limitation of this work was its cross-sectional nature, making causal interpretation of the observed associations difficult. A further investigation, including a control group (subjects not suffering from Covid-19) would then be necessary to validate the results observed.

The third limitation related to the scales we used to assess anxiety-depressive disorders and post-traumatic stress. Although the scales used were reliable, valid and easy to use, they were screening scales, which could lead to an overestimation of the disorders in the absence of an associated psychiatric interview, and given the social disadvantage.

3. Study strengths :

To our knowledge, there have been no published studies assessing the mental health of Covid-19 patients in Tunisia. Yet psychological well-being is essential to improving the quality of care. The studies found in the literature search focused on medical and paramedical staff, as well as the general population.

This work has enabled us to observe the absence of a screening policy for disorders psychiatric care for patients with Covid-19.

In the course of our work, we used scales translated and validated in Arabic. In this way, our patients had no difficulty in understanding and answering the various items.

4. Prevalence of depressive symptoms after Covid-19:

In our study, the prevalence of depression was 65.84%, with mild intensity in 44.16% of cases. Our result was higher, compared to a meta-analysis made between 2019 and August 2020 (8) encompassing 31 studies conducted on a population of 5153 patients and to other studies (Table XIV).

Furthermore, our results were comparable to those reported in the Middle Eastern series and two Greater Maghreb countries (Table XIV). This finding could be explained by cultural and environmental similarities.

Table XIV: Prevalence of depression in various studies by country :

Study	Country **Prevalence**	Year	Scale used	
Jiawen Deng et al. (Meta-analysis including 20 studies) (9)	China	2020	SDS PHQ-9 HADS-D SCL-90	45%
Claudio Liguori et al.(10)	Italy	2020	Interview, SNS	38%
Paz et al.(11)	Ecuador	2020	PHQ-9 ≥ 5	60%
Btiss	Morocco	2020	HADS	53%
Zarrouqet al (12)	Libya	2020	PHQ-2	50%
M. Elhadi et al (13)			DASS-21	59%
S. Sma et al (14)	Moy en orient	2020	DASS-21	67,1%
Ahmed Arafa et al (15)	Egypt	2020		
Our study	Tunisia	2021	PHQ-9	65,84%

SDS: standard deviation scores ; PHQ-9 :Patient health questionnaire-9 : ; HADS-D : Hospital Anxiety and Depression scale; SNS: swiss narcolepsy scale SCL-90 : **Symptom** Checklist-90-;DASS-21: Depression, Anxiety and Stress Scale - 21

In addition to methodological differences (scales used (16), sampling fluctuation (9)), the difference in our result compared with Western and Asian series may be due to other factors. Indeed, quarantine for a health crisis was a first for the majority of Tunisians; unlike other countries such as China, which has been confronted with previous epidemics such as Severe Acute Respiratory Syndrome (SARS) (17).

In addition, the difficulties of managing the pandemic (lack of materials and personal protective equipment, saturation of care services, periods of oxygen shortage) constituted additional sources of stress, which could increase the prevalence of depression under our skies, compared with the West (14). Finally, the majority of studies were carried out in the general population, whereas our study only included subjects with Covid-19. This population would be more likely to develop depression.

In fact, since ancient times, depression has been linked to infectious diseases such as Chlamydophila trachomatis, Borna's disease, varicella-zoster virus, herpes simplex 1 and Epstein-Barr (18). This link is thought to be related to the virus-induced inflammatory effect and cytokine storm (19) (20) (figure26). Peripheral cytokine release reaching the brain via humoral and neural pathways, and ensuring release by microglial cells, would induce neuronal damage and neurogenesis-like neuronal apoptosis linked to increased glutamatergic concentrations and decreased levels of altered BDNF.

What's more, the relationship between inflammation and depression is thought to be bidirectional. Thus, a depressive disorder would be associated with elevated levels of pro-inflammatory cytokines (21). In fact, psychological or physiological stress triggered the production of pro-inflammatory cytokines that activate IDO. This enzyme catalyzes the breakdown of tryptophan and is involved in the conversion of serotonin to kynurenine (KYN). KYN is subsequently metabolized into tryptophan catabolites such as neuroprotective kynurenic acid (KA) and neurotoxic quinolinic acid (QUIN). Increases in these two acids in the central and peripheral nervous systems have been associated with IFN-a-induced depression. In addition, activation of IDO leads to activation of glutamatergic receptors and reduced serotonin synthesis. Cellular damage induced by neurotoxic tryptophan and glutamate metabolites also increases the risk of depression, (22) , (23).

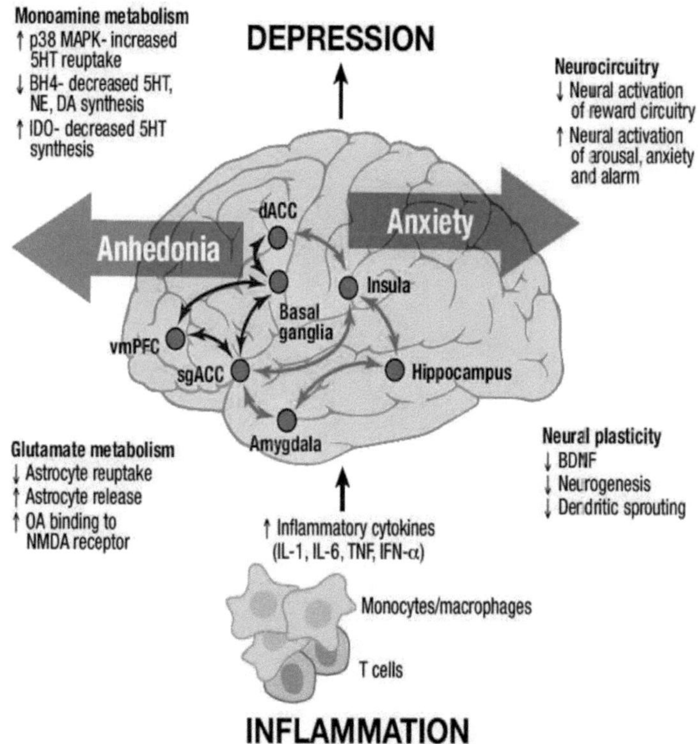

Figure Impact of inflammation on the brain and behavior

5HT, serotonin; BDNF, brain derived neurotrophic factor; BH4, tetrahydrobiopterin; DA, dopamine; dACC, dorsal anterior cingulate cortex; IDO, indoleamine 2,3 dioxygenase; IFN-interferon; IL, interleukin; MAPK, mitogen activated protein kinase; NE, norepinephrine; NMDA, N-methyl-D-aspartate; QA, quinolinic acid; sgACC, subgenual anterior cingulate cortex; TNF, tumor necrosis factor.

Figure 26: Link between depression and inflammation

5. Prevalence of anxiety symptomatology in post Covid-19:

In our study, the prevalence of anxiety symptoms was 96%, with moderate anxiety in 60% of cases. Our rate appears alarming. It was higher than those reported in the literature (Table XV).

Table XV: Prevalence of anxiety in different studies

Study used	Country	Year	Tool	**Préval** ence
Jiawen Deng et al (Meta analysis including 20 studies) (9)	China	2020	SAS GAD-7 HADS-A SAS SCL-90	48%
Liguori et al.(10)	Italy	2020	Interview	33%
Paz et al(11)	Equate ur	2020	GAD-7 ≥ 5	65%
B. Zarrouqet al.(12)	Morocco	2020	HADS	43%
M. Elhadi et al(13)	Libya	2020	GAD-7	51%
S. Sma, et al (14)	Middle East	2020	DASS-21	60%
A. Arafa et al (15)	Egypt	2020	DASS-21	53,3%
Our study	Tunisia	2021	GAD-7	96%

SDS: standard deviation scores ; HADS-A: Hospital Anxiety and Depression scale; SCL-90 : **Symptom** Checklist-90-;DASS-21: Depression, Anxiety and Stress Scale - 21

The link between anxiety and Covid-19 may be related to several factors. Firstly, Covid-19 has been associated with a great deal of uncertainty. Indeed, the variability of clinical presentations, the debated duration of the virus' persistence on surfaces, its incubation period and speed of progression would be a source of increased stress (24).

Secondly, at the start of the pandemic, our healthcare system was fragile in the face of this health crisis. This created a heightened sense of anxiety among people, aggravated by the fear of re-infection through frequent exposure to the virus (23). Finally, it has been reported that the lack of protective measures, the absence of vaccination and anxiety among medical and paramedical staff could be predictive factors of anxious symptomatology in patients (24).

Furthermore, the link between Covid-19 and anxiety could be explained by the association between respiratory symptomatology and anxiety symptomatology, more specifically panic disorder, which has been highlighted since the 1980s and even more so in the 1990s with Klein's theory (25). This was a hypothesis of the false alarm of suffocation. Our brains are sensitive to CO2, so lack of air leads to an increase in CO2 pressure, which is a panic-inducing stimulus leading to imminent suffocation.

Another neurobiological hypothesis was proposed by Deakin and Graeff in 1991, linking the cardiorespiratory and behavioral response to panicogens via central chemoreceptors such as the serotonergic neurons of the ventrolateral periaqueductal gray matter and the ventrolateral and dorsal raphe nucleus(26).

In summary, the pathophysiology of anxious symptomatology in respiratory infection remains poorly explained, but given its fairly high prevalence, especially in cases of mass hysteria (27), it is essential to detect it and take early action.

6. Link between anxiety-depressive symptomatology and the characteristics of the study population

6.1. Link between anxiety-depressive symptomatology and socio-demographic characteristics

6.1.1. Link between anxiety-depressive symptomatology and age :

We found a statistically significant relationship between anxiety-depressive symptomatology and age over 40 in univariate analysis (p=0.000) and linear regression.

This result was not in line with the findings of the various studies cited above. According to these studies, and as announced by the WHO (28), young people under the age of 35 were more likely to develop anxiety-depressive disorders. Young people had more access to news of the pandemic via social networks, and were more concerned about falling incomes and unemployment. These factors contribute to psychological distress (29).

However, the younger subjects took on more responsibilities, such as reorganizing and managing work, finding resources for their families, and providing help and advice to the youngsters, which presented a source of additional stress and thus explained our result.

6.1.2. Link between anxiety-depressive symptomatology and the genre

In our study, we found that men presented higher mean scores for depression (p=0.007) and anxiety (p=0.088). In multivariate analysis, we found a statistically significant association between gender and depression score (p=0.016).

These results differed from those reported in the literature (30). Women were found to bemore likely to develop anxiety-depressive symptomatology during the Covid-19 pandemic. Women had more risk factors for depression inherent in the increase in violence against them, especially during periods of confinement (31).

(12) and hormonal and sentimental changes (32).

Furthermore, in our study, the link between male gender and anxiety-depressive symptomatology could be due to the average age, which was 57 in our study. Indeed, from the age of 60 onwards, men and women had a similar prevalence of anxiety-depressive disorders (32)(33). Moreover, men were more likely to be affected by the virus, given the presence of the ACE2 protein in the testicles and not in the ovaries (34) (35). Men were also more likely to be hospitalized with severe forms of the disease, according to a Chinese study (36), and to have a less robust humeral and cellular response than women(37). As a result, they were at greater risk of developing anxiety-depressive disorders.

6.1.3. Link between anxiety-depressive symptomatology and the marital status :

In our study, married subjects had mean symptomatology scores of more anxiety-depressive than singles, with no statistically significant relationship.

This finding was consistent with the literature, where single status was considered a protective factor against the pandemic (38). Married subjects would have the anxiety of contaminating a family member, of feeling guilty especially as most people did not benefit from special accommodation during confinement.

6.1.4. Link between anxiety-depressive symptomatology and living area :

In our study, we found a statically significant association between urban dwelling area and mean depression and anxiety scores with $p=0.048$ and $p=0.005$ respectively.

This result was in line with the literature. A Chinese study showed that the prevalence of depression was 15.3% in urban areas and 12.4% in rural areas. Similarly, the prevalence of anxiety was 27.5% in urban areas and 23.2% in rural areas (39).

In fact, according to a Chinese review of 4607 patients carried out in March 2020, living in an urban area was associated with other factors such as attitudes taken during periods of confinement and a drop in socio-economic level; this would increase the prevalence of anxiety-depressive disorder (40) (41).

In addition, the high population density in urban areas potentially increases the risk of the virus spreading (42). Thus, residents of these areas could experience more stressors due to a higher perceived risk of COVID-19 infection. In addition, strategies of social distancing could lead to loneliness and isolation, precipitating depression and anxiety. Rural residents, on the other hand, lived in more spacious areas and would therefore be less affected by social distancing and quarantine measures. Finally, residents of these isolated areas tended to receive less information about the pandemic due to limited media sources, which would lessen the adverse effects on mental health.

6.1.5. Link between anxiety-depressive symptomatology and level of education :

In our study, mean depression and anxiety scores were statistically correlated with illiterate subjects with p= 0.032 and p=0.006 respectively, with no prior linear relationship. These results were in line with those of a meta-analysis encompassing 89 studies (43).

Illiterate subjects tend to seek information via unofficial sources, at the risk of receiving false information. In our study, 66.6% used social networks. According to the WHO report, the infodemia that has accompanied this pandemic has increased stress and harmed people's mental and physical health. It also increased stigmatization and led to non-compliance with public health measures (44).

With this in mind, it would be a good idea to create action plans to disseminate accurate information to people, taking into account their level of education.

6.2. Link between anxiety-depressive symptomatology and clinical and therapeutic features :

6.2.1. Link between anxiety-depressive symptomatology and the after-effects of Covid-19 :

In our study, we found a statistically significant relationship between mean depression and anxiety scores and disease sequelae in univariate analysis with p<0.001 and p=0.001 respectively.

These sequelae are part of the "long Covid", a complex, multifactorial disease describing the residual effects of acute SARS-CoV-2 infection (45).

A comparative study between two Japanese and Swedish populations, carried out on 763 patients between March and June 2021, had concluded that the presence of Covid-19 sequelae doubled the risk of having a psychiatric disorder (46).

The anxiety-depressive disorder could manifest as dyspnoea (47), headaches, memory disorders (48) or digestive disorders (49). These symptoms were found to be sequelae of Sars cov2 disease both in our study and in the literature (50) (51). However, the pathophysiology remains poorly understood. The interactions between anxiety-depressive symptomatology and physical symptoms such as pain and asthenia frequently found in post-covid are complex (52). On the one hand, physical symptoms could be attributable to viral infections or to the host immune response (53); this has been described in past pandemics: SARS-CoV-1, MERS-CoV (54) (55). On the other hand, physical sequelae may be related to the somatization phenomenon described during depression (56). This phenomenon, expressed by somatic signs such as asthenia, is the body's response to protect itself against psychic pressures and tensions. This phenomenon is seen as the body's cry for psychological help (57).

6.2.2. Link between anxiety-depressive symptomatology and the use of respiratory assistance :

In our work, we found no association between the use of respiratory assistance and the PHQ-9 and GAD-7 scores.

This was not consistent with the literature. Indeed, in a study of 163 Italian patients, anxiety-depressive disorder was significantly greater in subjects who required artificial ventilation, with p= 0.017 (58). Similarly, in a study by Lizé et al, 50% of patients hospitalized in the ICU and requiring intubation presented more depressive symptoms and insomnia (59). This finding may be related to the presence of lung lesions and the drop in oxygen saturation (60).

The difference in our result could be explained firstly by the difference inage compared with the other studies, and secondly by the low prevalence of intubated patients hospitalized in the intensive care setting in our case.

6.2.3. Link between anxiety-depressive symptomatology and length of time off work :

We found a statistically significant link between the duration of work stoppage and the mean depression score (p=0.031) on the one hand, and the mean anxiety score (p=0.002) on the other.

In our context, work stoppage was synonymous with health confinement. Studies have shown that the longer the period of leave, the greater the risk of psychological damage (61). In this context, it has been reported in France that a fairly long period of leave degrades mental health by 26% (62). Furthermore, a Chinese study of 369 patients concluded that mental health and satisfaction levels were poorer for non-workers than for workers (63) (64).

The link between anxiety-depressive symptomatology and work stoppage could be explained by the fear of reinfection, given the lack of protective means, as explained in M.-F. Richard's study (61). What's more, when isolation is carried out at home, the fear of infecting close relatives is always present (65),(66), which constitutes an additional stress factor.

6.3. Link between anxiety-depressive symptomatology and stigmatization :

We found a statistically significant association between the anxiety symptoms and feelings of stigmatization with p=0.022.

This finding was similar to that reported in the literature. Indeed, since the outbreak of the pandemic, there has been a negative perception of those infected with the disease. Covid-19 patients were acc u49 sed to be ignorant and negligent, and therefore held responsible for contracting the virus. They were considered active propagators of the virus (67). As a result, the fear of contracting the disease was seen as one of the main precursors to the stigmatization of infected people (68). Discriminatory reactions against the stigmatized have also been a cause for concern in the context of long-standing epidemics such as Severe Acute Respiratory Syndrome (SARS) (69) and H5N1 (70) . These factors are said to be the source of social rejection and have repercussions on the physical and psychological health and well-being of the stigmatized.

6.4. Link between anxiety-depressive symptomatology and the need to psychological support :

In our study, people who expressed a need for psychological support had significantly higher mean scores for depression (p=0.002) and anxiety (p=0.005).

These results were consistent with the literature. Patients who reported a need for psychological support were more likely to develop anxiety-depressive symptoms (71). This suffering could be due to a number of factors, such as confinement, isolation and feelings of loneliness (71). A study published by Unicef found that 24% of people felt isolated and didn't know where to turn for help during Covid-19 (72). Loneliness was an aggravating factor in mental health, as mentioned in a Spanish study of 3,480 patients carried out in 2020 (73), or during past pandemics (74). On the other hand, having a family, roommate or life partner was an essential factor in coping with the pandemic and meeting psychological needs (75) (73).

To meet this need for help, public health in France, for example, has launched platforms with a space dedicated to mental health (76) to help people access information and respond to their suffering (77). Teleconsultations have also been set up, as on the https://covidecoute.org/

website. Telemedicine has proved its usefulness in mental health for several years now (78). For example, the WHO has created an application that allows users to answer questions while sending a "hello" message to 0041718931892 on What's App to activate the conversation (79). In Tunisia, the University of Tunis, in collaboration with the psychologists' office, launched a hotline fstudents during a pandemic (80). The aim of these different strategies was to disseminate accurate information and create a favorable climate for psychological support, in order to mitigate the impact of psychological distress.

6.5. Link between anxiety-depressive symptomatology and behavior during the pandemic :

In our study, we found no significant relationship between anxiety-depressive symptomatology and information source. Furthermore, 66.6% of patients sought information via social networks and multimidia, which is in line with the literature. Indeed, despite the fact that the world has previously experienced devastating pandemics in economic and human terms (many deaths), this pandemic was associated with a veritable infodemia. The rapid sharing of misrepresentations, misinformation and magic remedies was detrimental to mental health, increasing the risk of anxiety-depressive disorders (81).

7. Prevalence of post-traumatic stress symptomatology and COVID-19 :

In our study, 52.2% of patients had post-traumatic stress disorder.
traumatic.

In the past, the prevalence of PTSD was estimated at between one and 10% in the general population (82). During the COVID-19 pandemic, the prevalence of PTSD increased according to several studies carried out worldwide (Table XVI).

Table XVI: Prevalence of PTSD by country :

Study	**Country**	**Screening tool**	**Number of inhabitants**	**Prev alence**
Giuseppe Forte et al(84)	Italy	COVI D-19PTSD	2286	29, 5%
Halah Bin Helayel et al(85)	Saudi Arabia	IES-R	111	28, 8%
N. Np et al(86)	Afri than south	IES-R	489	35, 4%
P. C. Mboua, et al (87)	Cameroon	IES-R	384	70, 7%

Fekih Romdhane et al (83)	Tunisia	IES-R	603	33%
Our study	Tunisia	IES-R	120	52, 2%

IES- : IMPACT OF EVENTS SCALE-REVISED; COVID-19 PTSD: COVID-19 POST TRAUMATIC STRESS DISORDER QUESTIONNAIRE

In addition, a meta-analysis including 381 patients with covid-19 showed a prevalence of 30.2% (88). Furthermore, a review of the literature including 19 studies (89) (10 from China, two from Spain, two from Italy, one from Iran, one from the USA, one from Denmark, one from Turkey and one from Nepal) concluded that the prevalence of PTSD was 53.8%, which concurred with our result.

It has been pointed out that during any pandemic or natural disaster, the general population presents high prevalences of PTSD (90). The Covid-19 pandemic was a traumatic event. Indeed, people were exposed to violent images of overflowing health care services and processions of the dead in some countries. In addition, subjects were more exposed to potentially psycho-traumatic confrontations and stress, particularly as a result of confinement, new government measures and lack of information.

The higher rate of post-traumatic stress disorder in our study, compared with other studies, could be explained by the fact that our population was surveyed one month after the Covid infection, indicating a high impact of the trauma, and by our patients' poor psychological preparation for the various psycho-traumatic confrontations. The Jasmine Revolution in Tunisia increased the prevalence of PTSD from 1% to 27.1% (91) (92). However, this prevalence of PTSD should be treated with caution, as the identification of this disorder was based on a psychometric scale obtained by telephone call, rather than a clinical interview.

8. Link between post-traumatic stress symptomatology and the characteristics of the population :

8.1. Link between post-traumatic stress symptomatology and general characteristics of the population :

8.1.1. Link between the symptomatology of post and age:

In our study, IES-R scores were significantly higher in patients aged over 40 (p=0.000). Age was also an independent predictor of PTSD.

In Tunisia, a study of 157 patients at the FSI hospital in La Marsa in November 2021(93) showed that the prevalence of PTSD was more frequent in older patients (mean age 56.4 years); this was consistent with our study. On the other hand, age was not a predictor of PTSD in a Korean study of 107 patients (94). In other studies, younger subjects were more likely to develop PTSD (88). Similarly, according to an online field study in the United States involving4909 participants, adolescents and elderly subjects with a somatic history were most likely to develop PTSD (95). Indeed, advanced age is considered a poor prognostic factor(96).

8.1.2. Relationship between post-traumatic stress symptomatology and gender :

In our study, men had a higher mean post-traumatic stress symptomatology score than women, but there was no statistically significant relationship.

The data in the literature are controversial. Some studies have shown that women are more likely to develop PTSD, while others have not (97) (98) (99). Although men are more likely to be exposed to trauma, women are at greater risk of developing post-traumatic stress symptoms, due to hormonal, socio-cultural and biological factors(100).

8.1.3. Relationship between post-traumatic stress symptomatology and marital status :

In our study, we found no link between the mean score of the
and martial status (p=0.583).
Single status was a protective factor for post-traumatic stress. Moreover, according to a meta-analysis, parenthood irrespective of marital status (married, widowed, divorced) was an additional stress factor in the prevalence of post-traumatic stress disorder (90).

8.1.4. Relationship between post-traumatic stress symptomatology and level of education :

With regard to level of education, we found a statistically significant association between illiteracy and IES-R score (p=0.009). Our finding was in line with the literature (101) (102). A Belgian study assessing peri-traumatic factors during the Covid 19 pandemic showed that education was a protective factor against psychological distress (103).

The link found in our study could be related to the source of information. Subjects tend to seek information via their social networks. However, the pandemic was accompanied by misinformation and misrepresentation, leading to infodemia (104). The latter was a source of added stress and increased the risk of psychological distress.

8.2. Relationship between post-traumatic stress symptomatology and clinical features :

8.2.1. Link between post-traumatic stress symptomatology and the need for respiratory assistance:

In our work, the use of respiratory assistance was significantly associated with the IES-R score in univariate (p=0.028) and multivariate (p=0.012) analysis.

Our findings were in line with the literature. According to a meta-analysis, respiratory assistance was a pre-trauma vulnerability factor predisposing to PTSD. Indeed, among subjects requiring hospitalization in an intensive care or resuscitation unit, 24% of patients had developed PTSD at one month post-Covid according to 36 cohorts encompassing 4200 participants (105). Similarly, a Tunisian study found that 36% of patients requiring high-flow oxygen therapy developed PTSD (93). An increased risk of PTSD has been observed in survivors of MERS and SARS in the past, and of COVID-19 in the present, particularly in patients following a hospital course, including intensive care inpatients, mechanically ventilated and intubated patients (106).

The association between this factor and PTSD could be explained in part by the anxiety-provoking environmental factors of the intensive care setting, namely the loss of spatio-temporal reference points, as well as the loss of autonomy, noise, light, equipment, isolation and limited, difficult interactions. Thus, frightening memories during the stay and the feeling of pejorative emotions when recalling the illness could be associated with greater psycho-traumatic symptomatology.

8.2.2. Link between post-traumatic stress symptomatology and duration of work stoppage :

In our study, patients who had taken time off work had presented more post-traumatic stress symptoms (p=0.014).

We found no studies associating this factor with a greater risk of PTSD. On the other hand, an article published by the Institut national de recherche et de sécurité in France highlighted the fact that around 14% of work stoppages were due to post-covid-19 psychosocial risks. In fact, according to Malakoff Humanis (107), covid-19 had become the leading cause of work stoppage. The ten days' absence from work was associated with compulsory quarantine for subjects testing positive. This quarantine was said to be a source of boredom and frustration, and was described by most subjects as a distressing, even traumatic experience (108).

8.3. Link between post-traumatic stress symptomatology and the need for psychological support :

We found that patients who expressed a need for psychological support showed greater post-traumatic symptomatology (p=0.005).

This finding was consistent with the literature. In America, according to an over-cited study (109), most respondents who had received social support had low levels of PTSD. This finding further underlines the need to facilitate access to psychological and mental health support structures, and to monitor patients during and after their hospital stay in the short, medium and long term. In France, the Haute Autorité de Santé has insisted on the need for post-hospital psychiatric follow-up in search of PTSD symptoms (110). In some Scandinavian countries, a diary is used to monitor admitted patients. This diary makes it possible to maintain a presence with the patient and give a human dimension to care and the individual, and consequently presents a protective effect against PTSD (111).

9. Comorbidity of anxiety-depressive and post-traumatic stress symptoms traumatic

We found a statistically significant relationship between the presence of post-traumatic stress symptomatology and anxiety-depressive symptomatology (p=0.004). According to Breslau et al, the risk of PTSD after a traumatic event was three times higher in the presence of pre-existing depression; PTSD increased the risk of a first depression after such an event (112). Depressive disorders could be present during, after or before the traumatic event. Thus, on the one hand, depression represented an evolving modality of a genuine psycho-traumatic sequel, and on the other a risk factor, comorbid or excluding PTSD.

Several studies have examined the association between depression and PTSD, with controversial results. For some, this comorbidity was an artifact of overlapping symptoms. Indeed, these disorders shared certain symptoms such as sleep disturbance, anhedonia, feelings of guilt and difficulty concentrating (113). Thus, changes in the way PTSD was conceptualized in the DSM had significantly affected the rate of association over time (113). Other studies had suggested that patients with PTSD and depressive symptomatology presented clinically and biologically different symptoms from those with depressive symptomatology or PTSD separately (114). Biologically, lower alpha-2 adrenergic receptor availability and higher plasma tyrosine affinity in the brain were associated with this comorbidity, but not with PTSD alone (114). Moreover, cerebrospinal fluid homovanillic acid was higher in depressed subjects with comorbid PTSD than in those with PTSD or isolated depressive disorder (114). On a molecular level, methylation of the glucocorticoid receptor gene was less frequent in those with PTSD alone, compared with those with comorbid PTSD and depression(115).

In short, the explanation for this comorbidity remains difficult but important to consider. Indeed, the association of these two disorders has been correlated with more severe symptomatology and poorer prognosis than each disorder in isolation (116) (117).

10. Recommendations

Our work has highlighted the high prevalence of anxiety-depressive symptomatology and post-traumatic stress in subjects suffering from Covid-19. Indeed, the Covid-19 pandemic has been a source of psychological distress. Consequently, international and national recommendations have been drawn up to promote mental health among the general population (120). Thus, it has been recommended to:

- physical activity
- maintain sleep hygiene,
- reduce exposure to screens and use reliable sources of information
- maintain links and communication with loved ones).

Specific recommendations have also been drawn up for covid-19 patients. In this context, the WHO has strongly recommended the provision of psychosocial support (28). For hospitalized patients, psychological support provided by psychologists working in somatic care departments has been recommended; with particular attention to patients who have had a stay in intensive care and/or have required respiratory assistance.

In addition, the use of new electronic screening tools in the context of the Covid-19 pandemic was highlighted as a means of identifying mental health problems at an early stage and intervening in time.

In France, the PSYCOVID-19 service has been set up for anyone needing to share their experiences and concerns (64). In Tunisia, a toll-free number **80 105 050** has been set up by psychologists and doctors (119).

In practice :

For people with Covid-19, we recommend:

- Informing and directing people with Covid-19 to the resources available to them (INEAS guide, helpline, international recommendations)

- Raise awareness among somatic healthcare staff of the impact of the pandemic on mental health, and provide them with screening scales for the most common psychiatric disorders.

- Systematically screen Covid-19 patients for the most common disorders: depression, anxiety and post-traumatic stress. Screening could be staggered according to the phases of the pandemic (during, in the immediate aftermath and late). Priority would be given to the most vulnerable patients, in particular the elderly, males and those requiring respiratory assistance or with more comorbidities.

- Refer patients in distress to individual specialist consultations when necessary.

"as this is the third year of the pandemic, increased clinical vigilance of mental health issues for patients with severe Covid-19 infection, and follow-up studies beyond the first year after infection are important to ensure timely access to care" as mentioned by public health France **(121)**

CONCLUSIONS

In December 2019, the emergence of a new form of coronavirus (Sars-Cov2) created worldwide confusion. In March 2020, Covid-19 was declared a pandemic by the WHO. This situation was thus a source of psychological distress and stress, with an immediate and significant impact on mental health in the general population, highlighted by an abundant literature. However, work on these disorders in subjects suffering from COVID-19 remains limited.

The aim of our work was to assess the prevalence of post-traumatic stress and anxiety-depressive disorders in the general population with Covid-19, as well as the sociodemographic and clinical factors associated with these disorders.

To this end, we conducted a descriptive and analytical cross-sectional study in the emergency department of La Rabta University Hospital in Tunis over a six-month period between January and June 2021.

We included subjects aged at least 18 and subjects who had contacted Covid 19 at least 1 month ago. Children and adolescents under 18 years of age, subjects whose COVID-19 infection was less than one month old, those with sensory deficits and those with cognitive deficits that might interfere with the evaluation were not included.

We excluded subjects who had interrupted the evaluation and those who had not completed all the scales proposed for evaluation or whose forms were unusable.

We collected sociodemographic and clinical characteristics related to Covid- 19.

We collected epidemiological and clinical data relating to COvid-19 infection.

We assessed attitudes related to the pandemic, i.e. sources of information about the epidemic, attitudes adopted to prevent infection by the Sars cov2 virus, attitudes adopted in the event of a psychological complaint during the epidemic, recourse to psychological support and/or psychiatric consultation since the start of the epidemic.

We used the Patient Health Questionnaire (PHQ-9), Generalized Anxiety Disorder 7 (GAD-7) and Event Impact Scale-Revised (ES-R) in their Arabic versions to assess depressive, anxiety and post-traumatic stress symptomatology respectively.

A total of 120 participants were interviewed. The median age of the participants was 57, with extremes ranging from 19 to 82. Over half the participants (53.3%) were male, with a sex ratio equal to 1.14. Fifty-seven percent of participants (57%) had a somatic history. Nine participants (7.5%) had previously consulted a psychiatrist or psychologist.

Concerning covid-19 infection, the most common reason for consultation was dyspnea (n=78; 65%).

We noted a depressive, anxious and post-traumatic stress symptomatology in respectively 65.84%, 96% and 52.2% of our patients.

In univariate analysis, we found a statistically significant association between depressive symptomatology and the following parameters: age over 40 ($p=0.000$), male gender ($p=0.007$), being illiterate ($p=0.032$), living in an urban area($p=0.048$), having sequelae of the disease ($p<0.001$), having been off work for more than 15 days ($p=0.031$) and having expressed a need for psychological support $p=0.002$.

In linear regression, age and gender were the independent predictors of depressive symptomatology, with $p<0.001$ and $p=0.016$ respectively.

In univariate analysis, we found a statistically significant association between anxious symptomatology and the following variables: age over 40 ($p=0.000$), level of education($p=0.006$), living area ($p=0.005$), being hospitalized ($p=0.006$), having sequelae of the disease ($p=0.001$), feeling stigmatized ($p=0.022$), length of time off work ($p=0.002$) and having expressed the need for psychological support ($p=0.005$).

In linear regression, age over 40 was the only independent predictor of this symptomatology with $p<0.001$.

The IES-R score was significantly higher in participants aged over 40 ($p=0.000$). The score was low among illiterates ($p=0.009$).

The IES-R score was significantly higher among patients who expressed a need for psychological support ($p=0.005$), as well as those who had been discharged for more than 15 days ($p=0.014$).

In linear regression, age and use of respiratory assistance were the independent predictors of this disorder, with $p<0.001$ and $p=0.012$ respectively.

Our results were largely in line with the literature, highlighting the impact of the pandemic on the mental health of Covid-19 patients.

Specific measures are aimed at this population, in particular the elderly, males and those who have required respiratory assistance, to improve their psychological well-being and intervene in time in the event of psychological distress.

References :

1. WHO Declares COVID-19 a Pandemic - PubMed [Internet]. [cited August 14
2022]. Available at: https://pubmed.ncbi.nlm.nih.gov/32191675/

2. Pablo GS de, Vaquerizo-Serrano J, Catalan A, Arango C, Moreno C, Ferre F, et al. Impact of coronavirus syndromes on physical and mental health of health care workers: Systematic review and meta-analysis. Journal of Affective Disorders [Internet]. Oct 10, 2020 [cited June 28, 2022];275:48. Available from: https://www.ncbi.nlm.nih.gov/pmc/articles/PMC7314697/

3. T W, X J, H S, J N, X Y, J X, et al. Prevalence of mental health problems during the COVID-19 pandemic: A systematic review and meta-analysis. Journal of affective disorders [Internet]. Feb 15, 2021 [cited Aug 14, 2022];281. Available from: https://pubmed.ncbi.nlm.nih.gov/33310451/

4. Cases of anxiety and depression up 25% worldwide due to COVID-19 pandemic [Internet]. [cited March 31, 2022]. Available from : https://www.who.int/fr/news/item/02-03-2022-covid-19- pandemic-triggers-25-increase-in-prevalence-of-anxiety-and-depression- worldwide

5. K K, Rl S, Jb W. The PHQ-9: validity of a brief depression severity measure. Journal of general internal medicine [Internet]. 2001 Sep [cited 2022 Jul 3];16(9). Available from: https://pubmed.ncbi.nlm.nih.gov/11556941/

6. As T, S T, Gj A, Sh AM, S AM, Us A, et al. Development and validation of Arabic version of the Hospital Anxiety and Depression Scale. Saudi journal of anaesthesia [Internet]. may 2017 [cited 3 Jul 2022];11(Suppl 1). Available from: https://pubmed.ncbi.nlm.nih.gov/28616000/

7. Ali AM, Al-Amer R, Kunugi H, Stanculescu E, Taha SM, Saleh MY, et al. The Arabic Version of the Impact of Event Scale-Revised: Psychometric Evaluation among Psychiatric Patients and the General Public within the Context of COVID-19 Outbreak and Quarantine as Collective Traumatic Events. 2022 [cited 3 Jul 2022]; Available from: https://dx.doi.org/10.3390/jpm12050681

8. Deng J, Zhou F, Hou W, Silver Z, Wong CY, Chang O, et al. The prevalence of depression, anxiety, and sleep disturbances in COVID-19 patients: a meta-analysis. Annals of the New York Academy of Sciences [Internet]. [cited 9 Apr 2022]; Available from: https://www.ncbi.nlm.nih.gov/pmc/articles/PMC7675607/

9. Deng J, Zhou F, Hou W, Silver Z, Wong CY, Chang O, et al. The prevalence of depression, anxiety, and sleep disturbances in COVID-19 patients: a meta-analysis. Ann NY Acad Sci [Internet]. feb 2021 [cited Apr 9, 2022];1486(1):90-111. Available from: https://onlinelibrary.wiley.com/doi/10.1111/nyas.14506

10. C L, M P, M S, L S, N C, M I, et al. Subjective neurological symptoms frequently occur in patients with SARS-CoV2 infection. Brain, behavior, and immunity [Internet]. aug 2020 [cited 9 Apr 2022];88. Available from: https://pubmed.ncbi.nlm.nih.gov/32416289/

11. Anxiety and depression in patients with confirmed and suspected COVID-. 19 in Ecuador - PubMed [Internet]. [cited 9 Apr 2022]. Available from: https://pubmed.ncbi.nlm.nih.gov/32609409/

12. B Z, N A, Je H, Ae A, S A, M O, et al. An investigation of the association between religious coping, fatigue, anxiety and depressive symptoms during the COVID-19 pandemic in Morocco: a web-based cross-sectional survey. BMC psychiatry [Internet]. 22 May 2021 [cited 10 Apr 2022];21(1). Available from: https://pubmed.ncbi.nlm.nih.gov/34022849/

13. Elhadi M, Alsoufi A, Msherghi A, Alshareea E, Ashini A, Nagib T, et al. Psychological Health, Sleep Quality, Behavior, and Internet Use Among People During the COVID-19 Pandemic: A Cross-Sectional Study. Front Psychiatry [Internet]. 2021 [cited Apr 12, 2022];0. Available from: https://www.frontiersin.org/articles/10.3389/fpsyt.2021.632496/full

14. Sma S, D M, Mfh Q, Mz A, S A. Prevalence, Psychological Responses and Associated Correlates of Depression, Anxiety and Stress in a Global Population, During the Coronavirus Disease (COVID-19) Pandemic. Community mental health journal [Internet]. jan 2021 [cited 9 Apr 2022];57(1). Available from: https://pubmed.ncbi.nlm.nih.gov/33108569/

15. A A, A M, L S, S S. Psychological Impacts of the COVID-19 Pandemic on the Public in Egypt. Community mental health journal [Internet]. jan 2021 [cited10

16. Deng J, Zhou F, Hou W, Silver Z, Wong CY, Chang O, et al. The prevalence of depression, anxiety, and sleep disturbances in COVID-19 patients: a meta-analysis. Annals of the New York Academy of Sciences [Internet]. [cited 9 Apr 2022]; Available from: https://www.ncbi.nlm.nih.gov/pmc/articles/PMC7675607/

17. Cherry JD. The chronology of the 2002-2003 SARS mini pandemic. Paediatric Respiratory Reviews [Internet]. Dec 2004 [cited 10 Apr 2022];5(4):262. Available from: https://www.ncbi.nlm.nih.gov/pmc/articles/PMC7106085/

18. Wang X, Zhang L, Lei Y, Liu X, Zhou X, Liu Y, et al. Meta-Analysis of Infectious Agents and Depression. Sci Rep [Internet]. 2014 March 31 [cited 2022 May 3];4(1):1-10. Available from: https://www.nature.com/articles/srep04530

19. R D, Jc O, Gg F, Rw J, Kw K. From inflammation to sickness and depression: when the immune system subjugates the brain. Nature reviews Neuroscience [Internet]. 2008 Jan [cited 2022 Jun 26];9(1). Available from: https://pubmed.ncbi.nlm.nih.gov/18073775/

20. Neurological effects of covid 19 (coronavirus) on the brain [Internet]. Brain Institute. [cited May 3 2022]. Available from: https://institutducerveau-icm.org/fr/covid-19-depression/

21. Frontiers | Involvement of Innate and Adaptive Immune Systems Alterations in the Pathophysiology and Treatment of Depression | Neuroscience [Internet]. [cited 3 May 2022]. Available from: https://www.frontiersin.org/articles/10.3389/fnins.2018.00547/full

22. Miller AH, Maletic V, Raison CL. Inflammation and Its Discontents: The Role of Cytokines in the Pathophysiology of Major Depression. Biological psychiatry [Internet]. May 5, 2009 [cited June 26, 2022];65(9):732. Available from: https://www.ncbi.nlm.nih.gov/pmc/articles/PMC2680424/

23. R M. Inflammation 2010: new adventures of an old flame. Cell [Internet]. 19mars2010 [cité26juin2022];140(6). Disponiblesur: https://pubmed.ncbi.nlm.nih.gov/20303867/

24. S E, R C, M T, H BA, M K, R W, et al. Professional quality of life and resilience strategies among Tunisian healthcare workers during the covid-19 pandemic. undefined [Internet]. 25 Apr 2022 [cited 28 Jun 2022]; Available from: https://europepmc.org/article/pmc/pmc9035357

25. Df K. False suffocation alarms, spontaneous panics, and related conditions. An integrative hypothesis. Archives of general psychiatry [Internet]. Apr 1993 [cited June 28, 2022];50(4). Available from: https://pubmed.ncbi.nlm.nih.gov/8466392/

26. The Deakin/Graeff hypothesis: focus on serotonergic inhibition of panic - PubMed [Internet]. [cited June 28 2022]. Available from: https://pubmed.ncbi.nlm.nih.gov/24661986/

27. Javelot H, Weiner L. Panic and the pandemic: a review of the literature on the links between panic disorder and the SARS-CoV-2 epidemic. L'Encephale [Internet]. June 2020 [cited June 28, 2022];46(3):S93. Available from: https://www.ncbi.nlm.nih.gov/pmc/articles/PMC7241353/

28. Cases of anxiety and depression up 25% worldwide due to COVID-19 pandemic [Internet]. [cited March 31, 2022]. Available from : https://www.who.int/fr/news/item/02-03-2022-covid-19- pandemic-triggers-25-increase-in-prevalence-of-anxiety-and-depression- worldwide

29. Wang C, Song W, Hu X, Yan S, Zhang X, Wang X, et al. Depressive, anxiety, and insomnia symptoms between population in quarantine and general population during the COVID-19 pandemic: a case-controlled study. BMC Psychiatry [Internet]. dec 2021 [cited 14 Apr 2022];21(1):1-9. Available from: https://bmcpsychiatry.biomedcentral.com/articles/10.1186/s12888-021- 03108-2

30. Pappa S, Ntella V, Giannakas T, Giannakoulis VG, Papoutsi E, Katsaounou
P. Prevalence of depression, anxiety, and insomnia among healthcare workers during the COVID-19 pandemic: A systematic review and meta- analysis. Brain, Behavior, and Immunity [Internet]. aug 2020 [cited 13 Apr 2022];88:901. Available from: https://www.ncbi.nlm.nih.gov/pmc/articles/PMC7206431/

31. M A, J B, C R, C H, S O, S H. Violence Against Women During COVID- 19 Pandemic. Journal of interpersonal violence [Internet]. Aug 3, 2021 [cited Apr 14, 2022]; Available from: https://pubmed.ncbi.nlm.nih.gov/33685271/

32. Albert PR. Why is depression more prevalent in women? Journal of Psychiatry & Neuroscience : JPN [Internet]. jul 2015 [cited 13 Apr 2022];40(4):219. Available from: https://www.ncbi.nlm.nih.gov/pmc/articles/PMC4478054/

33. P B, G D, R J, G L, T B, M F, et al. The influence of age and sex on the prevalence of depressive conditions: report from the National Survey of Psychiatric Morbidity. International review of psychiatry (Abingdon, England) [Internet]. May 2003 [cited 17 Apr 2022];15(1-2). Available from: https://pubmed.ncbi.nlm.nih.gov/12745313/

34. Shastri A, Wheat J, Agrawal S, Chaterjee N, Pradhan K, Goldfinger M, et al. Delayed clearance of SARS-CoV2 in male compared to female patients: High ACE2 expression in testes suggests possible existence of gender- specific viral reservoirs. medRxiv [Internet]. Apr 17, 2020 [cited May 2, 2022];2020.04.16.20060566. Disponible sur: https://www.medrxiv.org/content/10.1101/2020.04.16.20060566v1

35. Sama IE, Ravera A, Santema BT, van Goor H, ter Maaten JM, Cleland JGF, et al. Circulating plasma concentrations of angiotensin-converting enzyme 2 in men and women with heart failure and effects of renin-angiotensin-aldosterone inhibitors. Eur Heart J [Internet]. May 14, 2020 [cited May 2,

2022];41(19):1810-7. Available from: https://academic.oup.com/eurheartj/article/41/19/1810/5834647

36. Jin JM, Bai P, He W, Wu F, Liu XF, Han DM, et al. Gender Differences in Patients With COVID-19: Focus on Severity and Mortality. Front Public Health [Internet]. 2020 [cited May 2, 2022];0. Available from: https://www.frontiersin.org/articles/10.3389/fpubh.2020.00152/full

37. Doctissimo. Covid-19: are men more affected than women? [Internet]. Doctissimo. 2021 [cited May 2, 2022]. Available from: https://www.doctissimo.fr/sante/epidemie/coronavirus-chinois/Covid-19-hommes-plus-touches-que-les-femmes

38. El-Hage W, Hingray C, Lemogne C, Yrondi A, Brunault P, Bienvenu T, et al. Healthcare professionals facing the coronavirus disease (COVID-19) pandemic: what risks for their mental health? L'Encephale [Internet]. June 2020 [cited June 29, 2022];46(3):S73. Available from: https://www.ncbi.nlm.nih.gov/pmc/articles/PMC7174182/

39. Urban-rural disparities in mental health problems related to COVID-19 in China. General Hospital Psychiatry [Internet]. Mar 1, 2021 [cited Apr 22, 2022];69:119-20. Available from: https://www.sciencedirect.com/science/article/pii/S0163834320301122

40. Z N, Er L, Z Z, H W, H L, R S, et al. Response to the COVID-19 Outbreak in Urban Settings in China. Journal of urban health : bulletin of the New York Academy of Medicine [Internet]. feb 2021 [cited 20 Apr 2022];98(1). Available from: https://pubmed.ncbi.nlm.nih.gov/33258088/

41. S R, K M, T S, Ck E, M H, K G, et al. Depression and Anxiety During the COVID-19 Pandemic in an Urban, Low-Income Public University Sample. Journal of traumatic stress [Internet]. feb 2021 [cited 20 Apr 2022];34(1). Available from: https://pubmed.ncbi.nlm.nih.gov/33045107/

42. Delamater PL, Street EJ, Leslie TF, Yang YT, Jacobsen KH. Complexity of the Basic Reproduction Number (R0) - Volume 25, Number 1-January 2019 - Emerging Infectious Diseases journal - CDC. [cited 22 Apr 2022]; Available from: https://wwwnc.cdc.gov/eid/article/25/1/17-1901_article

43. The prevalence of depressive symptoms, anxiety symptoms and sleep disturbance in higher education students during the COVID-19 pandemic: A systematic review and meta-analysis. Psychiatry Research [Internet]. 1 Jul 2021 [cited 29 Jun 2022];301:113863. Available from: https://www.sciencedirect.com/science/article/pii/S0165178121001608

44. Infodemia management on COVID-19: Promoting healthy behaviors and

mitigating the harmful effects of the dissemination of false and misleading information [Internet]. [cited June 29 2022]. available at: https://www.who.int/fr/news/item/23-09-2020-managing-the-covid-19-infodemic-promoting-healthy-behaviours-and-mitigating-the-harm-from-misinformation-and-disinformation

45. Taribagil P, Creer D, Tahir H. 'Long COVID' syndrome. BMJ Case Rep. Apr 2021;14(4):e241485.

46. K M, S H, E S, A K, G A. Impact of post-COVID conditions on mental health: a cross-sectional study in Japan and Sweden. BMC psychiatry [Internet]. 4 Apr 2022 [cited 24 Apr 2022];22(1). Available from: https://pubmed.ncbi.nlm.nih.gov/35379224/

47. A P, Jj A, Cw L, Mg C. Heart rate and heart rate variability in panic, social anxiety, obsessive-compulsive, and generalized anxiety disorders at baseline and in response to relaxation and hyperventilation. International journal of psychophysiology : official journal of the International Organization of Psychophysiology [Internet]. jan 2013 [cited 23 Apr 2022];87(1). Available from: https://pubmed.ncbi.nlm.nih.gov/23107994/

48. D M, C S, P H, P S, A S. Anxiety disorders in headache patients in a specialised clinic: prevalence and symptoms in comparison to patients in a general neurological clinic. The journal of headache and pain [Internet]. 2011 Jun [cited 2022 Apr 23];12(3). Available from: https://pubmed.ncbi.nlm.nih.gov/21298462/

49. M M, K K, Rl S, Jb W, W H, B L. Gastrointestinal symptoms in primary care: prevalence and association with depression and anxiety. Journal of psychosomatic research [Internet]. 2008 Jun [cited 2022 Apr 23];64(6). Available from: https://pubmed.ncbi.nlm.nih.gov/18501261/

50. Avis de l'Académie : Les séquelles de la Covid-19 - Académie nationale de médecine | Une institution dans son temps [Internet]. [cited 24 Apr 2022]. Available from: https://www.academie-medecine.fr/avis-de-lacademie-les-sequelles-de-la-covid-19/

51. #. Covid sequelae: 60% of hospitalized patients present at least one symptom after 6 months [Internet]. Press room | Inserm. 2021 [cited Apr 24, 2022]. Available from: https://presse.inserm.fr/covid-longue-60- des-patients-hospitalized-present-at-least-one-symptom-after-6- months/42865/

52. Understanding anxiety-depressive syndrome - Inicea [Internet]. [cited 23 Apr 2022]. Available from: https://www.inicea.fr/trouble/les-troubles-de-lhumeur/pathologie/la-depression/comprendre-le-syndrome-anxio-depressif

53. Ea T, Jn K, S H. Are we facing a crashing wave of neuropsychiatric sequelae of COVID-19? Neuropsychiatric symptoms and potential immunologic mechanisms. Brain, behavior, and immunity [Internet]. july 2020 [cited 24 apr 2022];87. Available from: https://pubmed.ncbi.nlm.nih.gov/32298803/

54. L K, S M, M C, J Y, Y W, R L, et al. Impact on mental health and perceptions of psychological care among medical and nursing staff in Wuhan during the 2019 novel coronavirus disease outbreak: A cross- sectional study. Brain, behavior, and immunity [Internet]. july 2020 [cited 25 apr 2022];87. Available from: https://pubmed.ncbi.nlm.nih.gov/32240764/

55. Je K, Jh H, Ho K, Sh S, Ss P, Th P, et al. Neurological Complications during Treatment of Middle East Respiratory Syndrome. Journal of clinical neurology (Seoul, Korea) [Internet]. jul 2017 [cited 25 Apr 2022];13(3). Available from: https://pubmed.ncbi.nlm.nih.gov/28748673/

56. Kettani Z. Somatization scale: differentiating between Covid-19 symptoms and somatization in young adults and elderly subjects. Npg [Internet]. dec 2020 [cited June 29, 2022];20(120):339. Available from: https://www.ncbi.nlm.nih.gov/pmc/articles/PMC7362795/

57. Kettani Z. Anxiety in young adults and elderly subjects during SARS-CoV2 pandemic-related containment. Npg [Internet]. dec 2020 [cited June 29, 2022];20(120):346. Available from: https://www.ncbi.nlm.nih.gov/pmc/articles/PMC7486034/

58. Post-traumatic stress disorder, depression and anxiety symptoms in COVID-19 outpatients with different levels of respiratory and ventilatory support in the acute phase undergoing three months follow up - PubMed [Internet]. [cited Aug 1, 2022]. Available at: https://pubmed.ncbi.nlm.nih.gov/35266658/

59. Patients on ventilators are at greater risk of mortality | Le Devoir [Internet]. [cited August 1, 2022]. Available from: https://content.jwplatform.com/previews/nGSyegM3-BQQIfVuL

60. Intersections between pneumonia, lowered oxygen saturation percentage and immune activation mediate depression, anxiety, and chronic fatigue syndrome-like symptoms due to COVID-19: A nomothetic network approach - PubMed [Internet]. [cited Aug 1, 2022]. Available from: https://pubmed.ncbi.nlm.nih.gov/34699853/

61. Richard MF. Epidemiological survey o f healthcare workers. reached by COVID-19 in spring 2020. 2020;76.

62. La-Croix.com. Confinement : les arrêts maladie de longue durée et les troubles psychologiques en augmentation [Internet]. La Croix. 2020 [cited 29 Apr 2022]. Available from: https://www.la- croix.com/Economie/Confinement-arrets-maladie-longue-duree-troubles- psychologiques-augmentation-2020-11-16-1201124894

63. Sx Z, Y W, A R, F W. Unprecedented disruption of lives and work: Health, distress and life satisfaction of working adults in China one month into the COVID-19 outbreak. Psychiatry research [Internet]. June 2020 [cited 28 Apr 2022];288. Available from: https://pubmed.ncbi.nlm.nih.gov/32283450/

64. Joboory SA, Monello F, Bouchard JP. PSYCOVID-19, a psychological support system in the fields of mental health, somatic care and medico-social care. Annales Medico-Psychologiques [Internet]. sept 2020 [cited 28 Apr 2022];178(7):747. Available from: https://www.ncbi.nlm.nih.gov/pmc/articles/PMC7315978/

65. Mengin A, Allé MC, Rolling J, Ligier F, Schroder C, Lalanne L, et al. Psychopathological consequences of confinement. L'Encéphale. June 2020;46(3):S43-52.

66. Markenson D, Woolf S, Redlener I, Reilly M. Disaster Medicine and Public Health Preparedness of Health Professions Students: A Multidisciplinary Assessment of Knowledge, Confidence, and Attitudes. Disaster med public health prep. oct 2013;7(5):499-506.

67. Bhanot D, Singh T, Verma SK, Sharad S. Stigma and Discrimination During COVID-19 Pandemic. Frontiers in Public Health [Internet]. 2020 [cited 29Jun 2022];8. Available from : https://www.ncbi.nlm.nih.gov/pmc/articles/PMC7874150/

68. DasV , Goffman E. Stigma , Contagion , Defect : Issues in the Anthropology of Public Health [Internet]. 2013 [cited June 29, 2022]. Disponiblesur: https://www.semanticscholar.org/paper/Stigma-%2C-Contagion-%2C-Defect-%3A-Issues-in-the-of-Das-Goffman/5113ba09191943a0234e59f5d5ef37b683d502a8

69. Person B, Sy F, Holton K, Govert B, Liang A, Ncid T, et al. Fear and Stigma: The Epidemic within the SARS Outbreak. Emerging Infectious Diseases [Internet]. Feb 2004 [cited June 29, 2022];10(2):358. Available from: https://www.ncbi.nlm.nih.gov/pmc/articles/PMC3322940/

70. R B, Pj B. Stigma in the time of influenza: social and institutional responses to pandemic emergencies. The Journal of infectious diseases [Internet]. 15 Feb 2008 [cited 29 Jun 2022];197 Suppl 1. Available from: https://pubmed.ncbi.nlm.nih.gov/18269326/

71. Bj S, Mh L. How the COVID-19 pandemic is focusing attention on loneliness and social isolation. Public health research & practice [Internet]. June 30, 2020 [cited 29Apr 2022];30(2). Available from: https://pubmed.ncbi.nlm.nih.gov/32601651/

72. "Living in Limbo: How coronavirus is impacting young people in Australia - UNICEF Australia [Internet]. [cited 29 Apr 2022]. Available from: https://www.unicef.org.au/our-work/unicef-in-emergencies/coronavirus- covid-19/living-in-limbo

73. Mental health consequences during the initial stage of the 2020 Coronavirus pandemic (COVID-19) in Spain. Brain, Behavior, and Immunity [Internet].
Jul 1, 2020 [cited Apr 30, 2022];87:172-6. Available from: https://www.sciencedirect.com/science/article/pii/S0889159120308126

74. B A, M M, Ma C. Loneliness, Sociodemographic and Mental Health Variables in Spanish Adults over 65 Years Old. The Spanish journal of psychology [Internet]. 10 Nov 2017 [cited 30 Apr 2022];20. Available from: https://pubmed.ncbi.nlm.nih.gov/29019303/

75. Te S. Health promoting effects of friends and family on health outcomes in older adults. American journal of health promotion : AJHP [Internet]. Aug 2000 [cited 29 Apr 2022];14(6). Available from: https://pubmed.ncbi.nlm.nih.gov/11067571/

76. COVID-19: taking care of your mental health during the epidemic [Internet]. [cited 1 May 2022]. Available from: https://www.santepubliquefrance.fr/maladies-et-traumatismes/maladies-et-infections-respiratoires/infection-a-coronavirus/articles/covid-19-prendre- soin-de-sa-santementale-pendant-l-epidemie

77. Psychic suffering and psychiatric disorders linked to the COVID-19 epidemic and difficulties of life in confinement: assessing them for better action [Internet]. [cited May 1, 2022]. Available from: https://www.santepubliquefrance.fr/presse/2020/souffrance-psychique-et-troubles-psychiatriques-lies-a-l-epidemie-de-covid-19-et-difficultes-de-la- vie-en-confinement-les-evaluer-pour-mieux-agir

78. Telepsychiatry: videoconferencing in the delivery of psychiatric care - PubMed [Internet]. [cited May 1, 2022]. Available from: https://pubmed.ncbi.nlm.nih.gov/23450286/

79. WHO's WhatsApp health alert service now available in French [Internet]. [cited 1 May 2022]. Available from: https://www.who.int/fr/news-room/feature-stories/detail/who-health-alert- brings-covid-19-facts-to-billions-

via-whatsapp

80. Meddeb A, Ayari F, Wesslati S, Abdennadher S. Coronavirus: advice from psychologists at the University of Tunis for coping with the crisis. :9.

81. Rathore FA, Farooq F. Information Overload and Infodemic in the COVID- 19 Pandemic. J Pak Med Assoc. May 2020;70(Suppl 3)(5):S162-5.

82. Traumatic events and Posttraumatic Stress Disorder: A review of the epidemiological literature. - Results of your search - Public health database [Internet]. [cited May 4 2022]. Available from: https://bdsp-ehesp.inist.fr/vibad/index.php?action=getRecordDetail&idt=217919

83. G F, F F, R T, M C. COVID-19 Pandemic in the Italian Population: Validation of a Post-Traumatic Stress Disorder Questionnaire and Prevalence of PTSD Symptomatology. International journal of environmental research and public health [Internet]. 6 Oct 2020 [cited 5 May 2022];17(11). Available from: https://pubmed.ncbi.nlm.nih.gov/32532077/

84. H BH, A A, Sk A, A A, R K, Sa AS. Quarantine-related traumatic stress, views, and experiences during the first wave of Coronavirus pandemic: A mixed-methods study among adults in Saudi Arabia. PloS one [Internet]. 13 Jan 2022 [cited 6 May 2022];17(1). Available from: https://pubmed.ncbi.nlm.nih.gov/35025910/

85. Np N, M ET, Raa Z, R OS, B B, Oc E, et al. Sex differences in the experience of COVID-19 post-traumatic stress symptoms by adults in South Africa. BMC psychiatry [Internet]. 4 Apr 2022 [cited 6 May 2022];22(1). Available from: https://pubmed.ncbi.nlm.nih.gov/35379197/

86. Mboua PC, Siakam C, Keubo FRN. Trauma and resilience associated with the COVID-19 pandemic in the cities of Bafoussam and Dschang, Cameroon. Annales Medico-Psychologiques [Internet]. nov 2021 [cited 22 May 2022];179(9):812. Available from: https://www.ncbi.nlm.nih.gov/pmc/articles/PMC8570645/

87. Fekih-Romdhane F, Ghrissi F, Abbassi B, Cherif W, Cheour M. Prevalence and predictors of PTSD during the COVID-19 pandemic: Findings from a Tunisian community sample. Psychiatry Research [Internet]. august 2020 [cited 10 may 2022];290:113131. Available from: https://www.ncbi.nlm.nih.gov/pmc/articles/PMC7255192/

88. D J, A C, Gd K, R B, F L, G S. Posttraumatic Stress Disorder in Patients After Severe COVID-19 Infection. JAMA psychiatry [Internet]. Jan 5, 2021 [cited May 7, 2022];78(5). Available from: https://pubmed.ncbi.nlm.nih.gov/33599709/

89. J X, O L, F N, Lmw L, H G, L P, et al. Impact of COVID-19 pandemic on mental health in the general population: A systematic review. Journal of affective disorders [Internet]. Jan 12, 2020 [cited May 6, 2022];277. Available from: https://pubmed.ncbi.nlm.nih.gov/32799105/

90. K Y, Ym G, L L, Yk S, Ss T, Yj W, et al. Prevalence of posttraumatic stress disorder after infectious disease pandemics in the twenty-first century, including COVID-19: a meta-analysis and systematic review. Molecular psychiatry [Internet]. sept 2021 [cited 2022 May 7];26(9). Available from: https://pubmed.ncbi.nlm.nih.gov/33542468/

91. Faten E, Sarah A, Rahma D, Sana E, Majda C. Mental disorders in Tunisia after Jasmin’s revolution. PSN [Internet]. 21 June 2017 [cited 9 May 2022];15(2):7-17. Available from: https://www.cairn.info/revue-psn-2017-2- page-7.htm

92. (PDF) Psychiatric disorders related to the events of the Tunisian revolution: about 107 cases managed at Razi Hospital outpatient clinic [Internet]. ResearchGate. [cited May 9, 2022]. Available from: https://www.researchgate.net/publication/246545591_Troubles_psychiatriques_in_relation_to_the_events_of_the_tunisian_revolution_a_propos_of_107_cases_taken_in_outpatient_consultations_at_Razi_hospital

93. Post-traumatic stress disorder after COVID-19 infection. Revue des Maladies Respiratoires Actualités [Internet]. 1 Jan 2022 [cited 22 May 2022];14(1):135. Available from: https://www.sciencedirect.com/science/article/pii/S1877120321008119

94. Incidence of Post-Traumatic Stress Disorder After Coronavirus Disease - PubMed [Internet]. [cited 2022 May 10]. Available from: https://pubmed.ncbi.nlm.nih.gov/33008081/

95. S M, T R, B T, L M, K K, E C, et al. The psychiatric sequelae of the COVID-19 pandemic in adolescents, adults, and health care workers. Depression and anxiety [Internet]. feb 2021 [cited May 22 2022];38(2). Available from: https://pubmed.ncbi.nlm.nih.gov/33368805/

96. Donamou J, Bangoura A, Camara LM, Camara D, Traoré DA, Abékan RJM, et al. Epidemiological and clinical characteristics of COVID-19 patients admitted to intensive care at Donka Hospital in Conakry, Guinea: descriptive study of the first 140 hospitalized cases. Anesthesia & Intensive Care [Internet]. March 2021 [cited June 29, 2022];7(2):102. Available from: https://www.ncbi.nlm.nih.gov/pmc/articles/PMC7859622/

97. C M, E R, S B, M C, S F, C N, et al. A Nationwide Survey of

Psychological Distress among Italian People during the COVID-19 Pandemic: Immediate Psychological Responses and Associated Factors. International journal of environmental research and public health [Internet]. Feb 5, 2020 [cited June 29, 2022];17(9). Available from: https://pubmed.ncbi.nlm.nih.gov/32370116/

98. Mz A, O A, Z A, S H, L S, A A. Epidemic of COVID-19 in China and associated Psychological Problems. Asian journal of psychiatry [Internet]. June 2020 [cited 29 June 2022];51. Available from: https://pubmed.ncbi.nlm.nih.gov/32315963/

99. C GS, B A, Má C, J S, A LG, C U, et al. Mental health consequences during the initial stage of the 2020 Coronavirus pandemic (COVID-19) in Spain. Brain, behavior, and immunity [Internet]. july 2020 [cited 29 june 2022];87. Available from: https://pubmed.ncbi.nlm.nih.gov/32405150/

100. W C, M M, W S, H B, J R. Gender difference, sex hormones, and immediate type hypersensitivity reactions. Allergy [Internet]. Nov 2008 [cited June 29, 2022];63(11). Available at: https://pubmed.ncbi.nlm.nih.gov/18925878/

101. Trauma and resilience associated with the COVID-19 pandemic in the cities of Bafoussam and Dschang, Cameroon. Annales Médico-psychologiques, revue psychiatrique [Internet]. Nov 1, 2021 [cited May 25, 2022];179(9):812-7. Available from: https://www.sciencedirect.com/science/article/pii/S0003448721001578

102. Qiu J, Shen B, Zhao M, Wang Z, Xie B, Xu Y. A nationwide survey of psychological distress among Chinese people in the COVID-19 epidemic: implications and policy recommendations. Gen Psych [Internet]. Apr 1, 2020 [cited May 25, 2022];33(2):e100213. Available from: https://gpsych.bmj.com/content/33/2/e100213

103. Beguin C. Trauma and Covid-19. Analysis of a frail population attending functional rehabilitation centers. :101.

104. Monnier A. Covid-19: from pandemic to infodemia and the hunt for fake news. Recherches & éducations [Internet]. May 11, 2020 [cited June 29, 2022];(HS). Available from: http://journals.openedition.org/rechercheseducations/9898

105. Vaiva PG. State of available knowledge and avenues of intervention. 2020;14.

106. Et K, Aj L. Post-traumatic stress disorder: A differential diagnostic consideration for COVID-19 survivors. The Clinical neuropsychologist

[Internet]. nov 2020 [cited 2022 May 24];34(7-8). Available from: https://pubmed.ncbi.nlm.nih.gov/32847484/

107. Coronavirus: psychosocial risks, the second most common reason for work stoppage in France [Internet]. Les Echos. 2020 [cited May 25, 2022]. Available from: https://www.lesechos.fr/economie-france/social/coronavirus-les-risques-psychosociaux-second-motif-darret-de-travail-en-france-1248678

108. Coronavirus: the psychological risks of confinement in 5 questions [Internet]. Les Echos. 2020 [cited 25 May 2022]. Available from: https://www.lesechos.fr/idees-debats/sciences-prospective/coronavirus-les-psychological-risks-of-confinement-in-5-questions-1189190

109. Ch L, E Z, Gtf W, S H, Hc H. Factors associated with depression, anxiety, and PTSD symptomatology during the COVID-19 pandemic: Clinical implications for U.S. young adult mental health. Psychiatry research [Internet]. August 2020 [cited 22 May 2022];290. Available from: https://pubmed.ncbi.nlm.nih.gov/32512357/

110. Haute Autorité de Santé - Prise en charge des patients post-COVID-19 en médecine physique et de réadaptation (MPR), en soins de suite et de réadaptation (SSR), et retour à domicile [Internet]. [cited 23 May 2022]. Available from: https://www.has-sante.fr/jcms/p_3179826/fr/prise-en-charge-des-patients-post-covid-19-en-medecine-physique-et-de- readaptation-mpr-en-soins-de-suite-et-de-readaptation-ssr-et-retour-a- domicile

111. Pa M, Rs K, M GO, A T, M R. The Effect of ICU Diaries on Psychological Outcomes and Quality of Life of Survivors of Critical Illness and Their Relatives: A Systematic Review and Meta-Analysis. Critical care medicine [Internet]. feb 2019 [cited May 23 2022];47(2). Available from: https://pubmed.ncbi.nlm.nih.gov/30431494/

112. N B, Gc D, El P, Lr S. A second look at comorbidity in victims of trauma: the posttraumatic stress disorder-major depression connection. Biological psychiatry [Internet]. Jan 11, 2000 [cited May 25, 2022];48(9). Available from: https://pubmed.ncbi.nlm.nih.gov/11074228/

113. Comorbidity between post-traumatic stress disorder and major depressive disorder: alternative explanations and treatment considerations - PMC [Internet]. [cited May 25 2022]. Available from: https://www.ncbi.nlm.nih.gov/pmc/articles/PMC4518698/

114. L S. The concept of post-traumatic mood disorder. Medical hypotheses [Internet]. 2005 [cited June 1, 2022];65(2). Available from: https://pubmed.ncbi.nlm.nih.gov/15922089/

115. R Y, Jd F, Lm B, C HH, A L, F D, et al. Lower methylation of glucocorticoid receptor gene promoter 1F in peripheral blood of veterans with posttraumatic stress disorder. Biological psychiatry [Internet]. Feb 15, 2015 [cited June 1, 2022];77(4). Available from: https://pubmed.ncbi.nlm.nih.gov/24661442/

116. Rc K, Cb N, Ka M, J L, M S, Dg B. Comorbidity of DSM-III-R major depressive disorder in the general population: results from the US National Comorbidity Survey. The British journal of psychiatry Supplement [Internet]. 1996 June [cited 2022 May 25];(30). Available from: https://pubmed.ncbi.nlm.nih.gov/8864145/

117. Mr J, Rb L. Comorbidity of major depression and panic disorder. Journal of clinical psychology [Internet]. feb 1998 [cited May 25, 2022];54(2). Available from: https://pubmed.ncbi.nlm.nih.gov/9467764/

118. gpc_covid_19_version_11_mai_2021.pdf [Internet]. [cited August 3, 2022].
Available on:
https://www.ineas.tn/sites/default/files/gpc_covid_19_version_11_mai_202 1.pdf

119. Coronavirus: The toll-free number dedicated is operational [Internet]. La Presse de Tunisie. 2020 [cited 1 May 2022]. Available from:
https://lapresse.tn/55650/coronavirus-le-numero-vert-consacre-a-laccompagnement-psychologique-des-citoyens-est-operationnel/

120. Mental health and COVID-19 [Internet]. [cited 2022 Aug 3]. Available from: https://www.santepubliquefrance.fr/dossiers/coronavirus-covid-19/enjeux- de-sante-dans-le-contexte-de-la-covid-19/articles/mental-health-and-covid-19

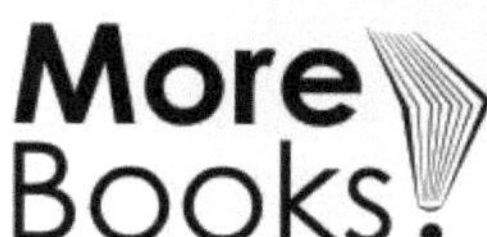

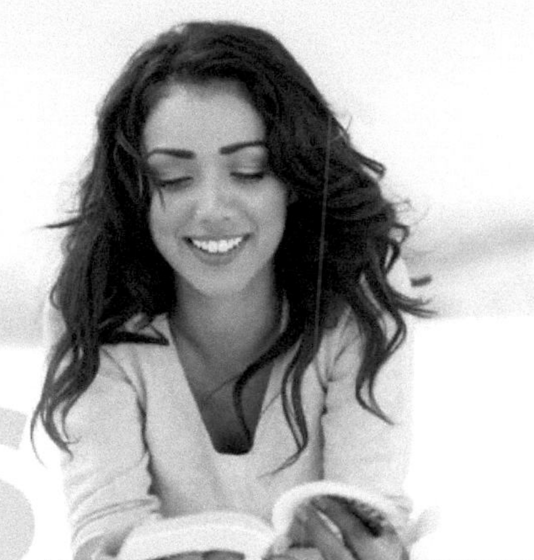

I want morebooks!

Buy your books fast and straightforward online - at one of world's fastest growing online book stores! Environmentally sound due to Print-on-Demand technologies.

Buy your books online at
www.morebooks.shop

Kaufen Sie Ihre Bücher schnell und unkompliziert online – auf einer der am schnellsten wachsenden Buchhandelsplattformen weltweit! Dank Print-On-Demand umwelt- und ressourcenschonend produzi ert.

Bücher schneller online kaufen
www.morebooks.shop

info@omniscriptum.com
www.omniscriptum.com

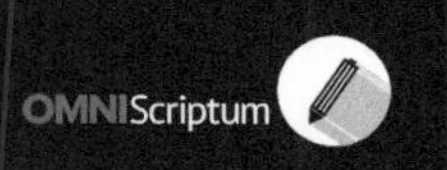

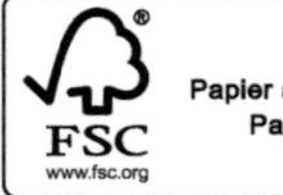

MIX
Papier aus verantwortungsvollen Quellen
Paper from responsible sources
FSC® C105338

Printed by Books on Demand GmbH, Norderstedt / Germany